Health at a Glance 2009

OECD INDICATORS

OECD

ORGANISATION FOR ECONOMIC CO-OPERATION AND DEVELOPMENT

The OECD is a unique forum where the governments of 30 democracies work together to address the economic, social and environmental challenges of globalisation. The OECD is also at the forefront of efforts to understand and to help governments respond to new developments and concerns, such as corporate governance, the information economy and the challenges of an ageing population. The Organisation provides a setting where governments can compare policy experiences, seek answers to common problems, identify good practice and work to co-ordinate domestic and international policies.

The OECD member countries are: Australia, Austria, Belgium, Canada, the Czech Republic, Denmark, Finland, France, Germany, Greece, Hungary, Iceland, Ireland, Italy, Japan, Korea, Luxembourg, Mexico, the Netherlands, New Zealand, Norway, Poland, Portugal, the Slovak Republic, Spain, Sweden, Switzerland, Turkey, the United Kingdom and the United States. The Commission of the European Communities takes part in the work of the OECD.

OECD Publishing disseminates widely the results of the Organisation's statistics gathering and research on economic, social and environmental issues, as well as the conventions, guidelines and standards agreed by its members.

This work is published on the responsibility of the Secretary-General of the OECD. The opinions expressed and arguments employed herein do not necessarily reflect the official views of the Organisation or of the governments of its member countries.

ISBN 978-92-64-06153-8 (print)
ISBN 978-92-64-07555-9 (PDF)
ISBN 978-92-64-07643-3 (HTML)
DOI 10.1787/health_glance-2009-en

Also available in French: *Panorama de la santé 2009 : Les indicateurs de l'OCDE*

Photo credits: Cover © Stockbyte/Fotosearch. Chapter 1: © Comstock/Jupiterimages. Chapter 2: © Comstock/Jupiterimages. Chapter 3: © Randy Faris/Corbis. Chapter 4: © Vincent Hazat/Photo Alto. Chapter 5: © CREATAS/Jupiterimages. Chapter 6: © onoky – Fotolia.com. Chapter 7: © Tetraimages/Inmagine.

Corrigenda to OECD publications may be found on line at: *www.oecd.org/publishing/corrigenda*.

Foreword

This latest edition of Health at a Glance illustrates the progress that has been made, both nationally and internationally, in measuring the performance of health systems. At their meeting in May 2004, Health Ministers asked the OECD to work with national administrations to improve the evidence base for comparing health system performance by: 1) ensuring that OECD Health Data would be timely and accurate; 2) continuing the implementation of health accounts to improve the availability and comparability of health expenditure and financing data; and 3) developing indicators of quality of care and health outcomes in collaboration with national experts. Substantial progress has been achieved in all of these areas, and this is reflected by the broader range of indicators of inputs, outputs and outcomes of health systems presented in this publication.

The production of Health at a Glance would not have been possible without the contribution of OECD Health Data National Correspondents, Health Accounts Experts, and experts involved in the Health Care Quality Indicators project. The OECD gratefully acknowledges their effort to supply most of the data and qualitative information contained in this publication. The OECD also acknowledges the contribution of other international organisations, especially the World Health Organisation and Eurostat, for sharing some of the data presented here, and the European Commission for supporting data development work in the area of health accounts and quality of care indicators.

This publication was prepared by a team from the OECD Health Division under the co-ordination of Gaétan Lafortune and Michael de Looper. Chapter 1 was prepared by Michael de Looper; Chapter 2 by Dominic Richardson, Franco Sassi, Michele Cecchini and Michael de Looper; Chapter 3 by Gaétan Lafortune, Rie Fujisawa and Jean-Christophe Dumont; Chapter 4 by Gaétan Lafortune, Valérie Paris, Gaëlle Balestat and Francis Notzon (from the National Centre for Health Statistics, United States); Chapter 5 by Ian Brownwood, Sandra Garcia Armesto, Niek Klazinga, Soeren Mattke (from Bain, United States) and Saskia Drösler (from Niederrhein University of Applied Sciences, Germany); Chapter 6 by Michael de Looper; and Chapter 7 by David Morgan, Roberto Astolfi and William Cave. All the figures were prepared by Gaëlle Balestat, with the exception of the figures for Chapter 5 which were prepared by Rie Fujisawa and Lihan Wei, and the figures for Chapter 7 which were prepared by David Morgan and Roberto Astolfi. This publication benefited from many comments and suggestions by Mark Pearson.

Table of Contents

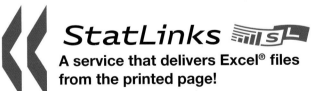

This book has...

StatLinks

A service that delivers Excel® files from the printed page!

Look for the *StatLinks* at the bottom right-hand corner of the tables or graphs in this book. To download the matching Excel® spreadsheet, just type the link into your Internet browser, starting with the ***http://dx.doi.org*** prefix.
If you're reading the PDF e-book edition, and your PC is connected to the Internet, simply click on the link. You'll find *StatLinks* appearing in more OECD books.

Introduction

H*ealth at a Glance* 2009 allows readers to compare health systems and their performance across a number of key dimensions, using a core set of indicators of health and health systems selected for their policy relevance and on the basis of the availability and comparability of the data.

The OECD has long been an international leader in the development of tools and collection of data for assessing the performance of health systems. OECD work to improve the comparability of health statistics goes back to the 1980s when efforts began to improve the comparability of health expenditure data, at a time when concerns emerged on rapidly rising health spending and the growing pressures on both public and private financing (OECD, 1985). The release of the manual, *A System of Health Accounts*, in 2000 provided a renewed impetus and key tool for the OECD to strengthen this effort to improve the comparability of health expenditure data across a larger group of countries, working in close collaboration with WHO and Eurostat.

While comparable data on health spending are necessary to assess the amount of financial resources that countries allocate to health, they are obviously not sufficient to assess the performance of health systems. The OECD effort to improve the comparability of health statistics was broadened to cover the supply and activities of health workers and physical resources in health care systems. Following the meeting of OECD Health Ministers in 2004, the OECD further extended its effort to assemble comparable data for assessing health system performance through developing and collecting a set of indicators to measure the quality of care and the outcomes of health interventions. In addition, initial work has been undertaken on a set of indicators related to access to care, another key objective of health systems across OECD countries. The OECD continues to work with experts in its member states and with other international organisations to fill gaps in the assessment and comparison of health system performance.

Policy, economic and social context

Beginning in the second half of 2008, OECD countries entered into a deep economic recession. The June 2009 OECD projections indicate that GDP may decline by about 4% in the OECD area in 2009, and unemployment rate is projected to reach about 10% of the labour force by the end of 2010 (OECD, 2009b).

Government budgets provide a very important cushion for economic activity in the downturn, mainly through automatic stabilisers and discretionary spending or tax reductions. However, the result has been a marked increase in government deficits. When the economic recovery is sufficiently firm, substantial reductions in budget deficits will be required in many countries. The extent of government spending reductions and/or tax increases will depend on the strength of the recovery and the size of the deficit and cumulative debt.

Given that health spending accounts for a high and growing share of public budgets, it will be hard to protect it from any general effort to control public spending during or after the recession. The extent to which public spending on health may be affected will depend on the relative priority allocated to health compared to other priorities. It will also depend on the extent to which public spending on health brings demonstrated benefits in terms of better health outcomes for the population. In a context of scarce public resources, there will be growing pressures on Health Ministries and health care providers to demonstrate efficiency (cost-effectiveness) in how resources are allocated and spent. Chapter 5 presents some of the progress achieved thus far in measuring quality of care and health outcomes across countries, while noting that the set of measures is still partial and further effort is needed to improve data comparability.

Structure of the publication

The framework underlying this publication allows for examining the performance of health care systems in the context of a broader view of public health (Figure 0.1). This framework is based on one that has been endorsed for the OECD Health Care Quality Indicators project (Kelley and Hurst, 2006; Arah *et al.*, 2006).

The framework highlights that the goal of health (care) systems is to improve the health status of the population. Many factors influence the health status of the population, including those falling outside health care systems, such as the social, economic and physical environment in which people live, and individual lifestyle and behavioural

Figure 0.1. **Conceptual framework for health system performance assessment**

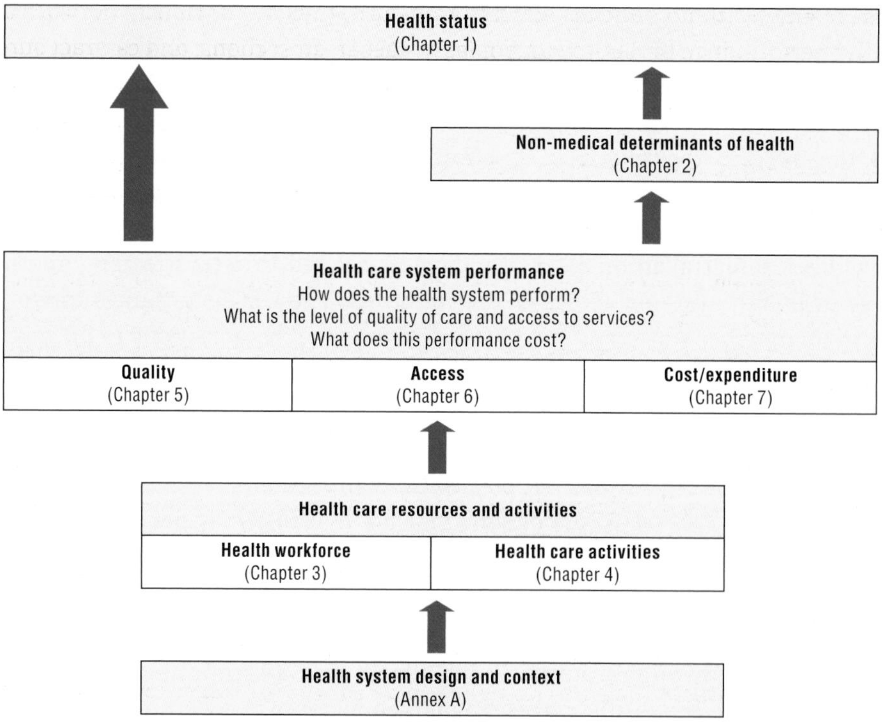

Source: Adaptation of the OECD (2006), "Conceptual Framework for the OECD Health Care Quality Indicators Project", OECD Health Working Paper, No. 23, OECD Publishing, Paris.

factors. The performance of health care systems also contributes to the health status of the population. This performance includes several dimensions, most notably the degree of access to care and the quality of care provided. Performance measurement also needs to take into account the financial resources required to achieve these access and quality goals. The performance of health systems depends on the people providing the services, and the training, technology and equipment that are at their disposal. Finally, a number of factors are related to health care system performance, such as the demographic, economic and social context, and the design of health systems.

Health at a Glance 2009 provides comparisons across OECD countries on each component of this framework. It is organised as follows:

- Chapter 1 on *Health Status* highlights large variations across countries in life expectancy, mortality and other measures of population health status.

- Chapter 2 on *Non-medical Determinants of Health* focuses on selected determinants related to modifiable lifestyles and behaviours. The chapter has been extended this year to cover risk or protective factors among children, such as nutrition habits, physical activity, smoking and alcohol drinking. These complement the set of adult risk factor indicators.

- Chapter 3 looks at the *Health Workforce*, the key actors in any health system. This new chapter provides information on the supply and remuneration of doctors and nurses, and recent trends on the international migration of doctors in OECD countries.

- Chapter 4 reviews a key set of *Health Care Activities*, both within and outside hospitals. It examines cross-country variations in the supply and use of medical technologies, such as medical resonance imaging (MRI) units and computed tomography (CT) scanners. It also looks at variations in the use of high-volume and high-cost procedures, such as coronary artery bypass graft and coronary angioplasty, caesarean sections, and cataract surgeries.

- Chapter 5 on *Quality of Care* provides comparisons on selected indicators of quality with respect to care for chronic conditions, mental disorders, cancers and communicable diseases. The measures include indicators of *process* of care that is recommended for certain population or patient groups to maximise desired outcomes, and key *outcomes* measures such as survival rates following heart attack, stroke and cancer.

- Chapter 6 is a new chapter on *Access to Care*, and aims to fill the gap in measuring this important dimension of health system performance. It begins with a limited number of indicators related to financial and geographic access. The intent is to expand this chapter in future editions, once further progress has been achieved in indicator development and data collection.

- Chapter 7 on *Health Expenditure and Financing* compares how much OECD countries spend on health, both overall and for different types of health services and goods. It also looks at how these health services and goods are paid for in different countries (*i.e.* the mix between public funding, private health insurance where it exists, and out-of-pocket payments by patients).

- Annex A provides some additional information on the demographic and economic context within which health systems operate, as well as some key characteristics of health system financing and delivery. This can assist readers in interpreting the indicators presented in the main body of the publication.

An increasing number of OECD countries are regularly publishing reports on different aspects of health and the performance of their health care systems. Examples of such national reports include *A Set of Performance Indicators across the Health and Aged Care System in Australia* (AIHW, 2008e), the *Dutch Health Care Performance Report* in the Netherlands (RIVM, 2008), *Quality and Efficiency in Swedish Health Care* in Sweden (Swedish Association of Local Authorities and Regions and National Board of Health and Welfare, 2008), and the *National Healthcare Quality Report* together with the *National Healthcare Disparities Report* in the United States (AHRQ, 2008a and 2008b). These national reports often focus on variations across different regions within the country. The Dutch performance report provides a good example of how such national reports may also be enriched by including international comparisons, to provide a broader perspective on the relative strengths and weaknesses of the national health system and identify potential areas for improvement.

Presentation of indicators

Each of the topics covered in the different chapters of this publication is presented over two pages. The first provides a brief commentary highlighting the key findings conveyed by the data, defines indicators and discloses any significant national variations from that definition which might affect data comparability. On the facing page is a set of figures. These figures typically show current levels of the indicator and, where possible, trends over time. In some cases, an additional figure relating the indicator to another variable is included. Where an OECD average is included in a figure, it is the unweighted average of the countries presented, unless otherwise specified in the accompanying notes.

Data limitations

Limitations in data comparability are indicated both in the text (in the box related to "Definition and deviations") as well as in footnotes to figures. Readers should exercise particular caution when considering time trends for Germany. Data for Germany up to 1990 generally refer to West Germany and data for subsequent years refer to unified Germany.

Readers interested in using the data presented in this publication for further analysis and research are encouraged to consult the full documentation of definitions, sources and methods contained in *OECD Health Data 2009*. This information is available free-of-charge at *www.oecd.org/health/healthdata*. *OECD Health Data 2009* can also be ordered online at SourceOECD (*www.sourceOECD.org*) or through the OECD's online bookshop (*www.oecd.org/bookshop*). Regarding Chapter 5 on *Quality of Care*, more information on definitions, sources and methods underlying the data is available at *www.oecd.org/health/hcqi*.

Population figures

The population figures presented in Annex A and used to calculate rates per capita throughout this publication come mainly from the OECD Labour Force Statistics Database (as at April 2009), and refer to mid-year estimates. Population estimates are subject to revision, so they may differ from the latest population figures released by national statistical offices of OECD member countries.

Note that some countries such as France, the United Kingdom and the United States have overseas colonies, protectorates and territories. These populations are generally excluded. The calculation of GDP per capita and other economic measures may, however, be based on a different population in these countries, depending on the data coverage.

Country codes (ISO codes)

Australia	AUS	Korea	KOR
Austria	AUT	Luxembourg	LUX
Belgium	BEL	Mexico	MEX
Canada	CAN	Netherlands	NLD
Czech Republic	CZE	New Zealand	NZL
Denmark	DNK	Norway	NOR
Finland	FIN	Poland	POL
France	FRA	Portugal	PRT
Germany	DEU	Slovak Republic	SVK
Greece	GRC	Spain	ESP
Hungary	HUN	Sweden	SWE
Iceland	ISL	Switzerland	CHE
Ireland	IRL	Turkey	TUR
Italy	ITA	United Kingdom	GBR
Japan	JPN	United States	USA

List of acronyms

AIDS	Acquired immunodeficiency syndrome
ALOS	Average length of stay
AMI	Acute myocardial infraction
ATC	Anatomic-therapeutic classification
BMI	Body Mass Index
CAD	Coronary artery disease
CAT (or CT)	Computed axial tomography
CHF	Congestive heart failure
COPD	Chronic obstructive pulmonary disease
DDD	Defined daily dose
DMFT	Decayed, missing or filled permanent teeth
EHR	Electronic health record
ESRF	End-stage renal failure
EU-SILC	European Union Statistics on Income and Living Conditions survey
GDP	Gross domestic product
GP	General practitioner
HBSC	Health Behavior in School-aged Children survey
HCQI	Health Care Quality Indicators (OECD Project)
HIV	Human immunodeficiency virus
ICHA	International Classification for Health Accounts
IHD	Ischemic heart disease
ISIC	International Standard Industrial Classification
MRI	Medical resonance imaging
PPP	Purchasing power parities
PSI	Patient safety indicators
PYLL	Potential years of life lost
SHA	System of Health Accounts
SIDS	Sudden infant death syndrome
UPI	Unique patient identifiers

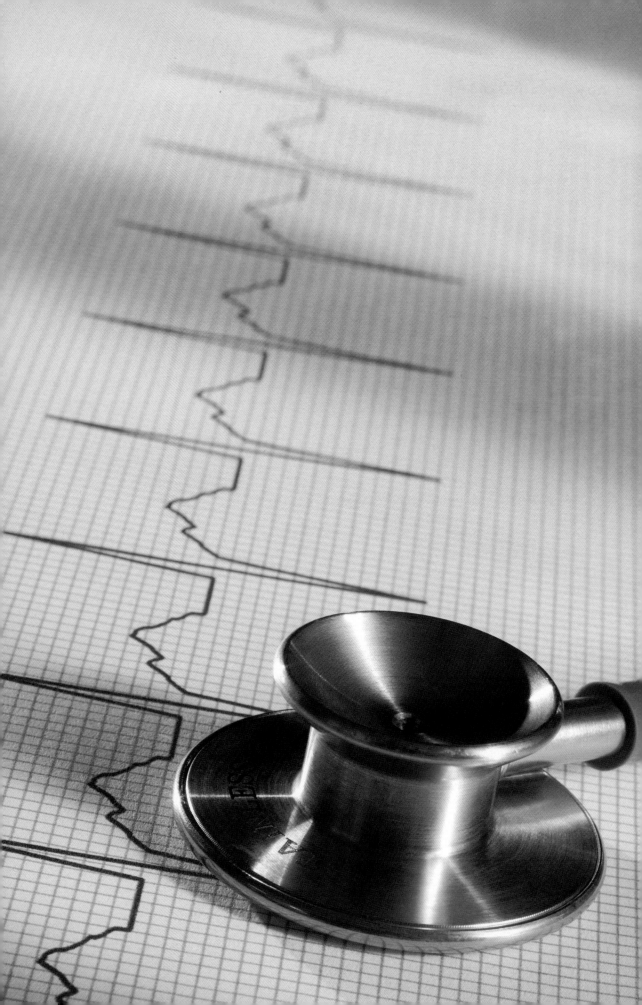

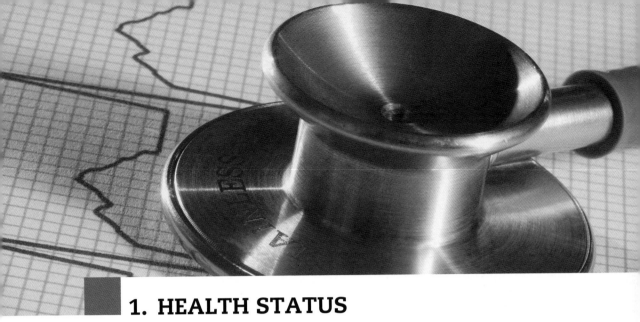

1. HEALTH STATUS

Life expectancy at birth has continued to increase remarkably in OECD countries, reflecting sharp reductions in mortality rates at all ages. These gains in longevity can be attributed to a number of factors, including rising living standards, improved lifestyle and better education, as well as greater access to quality health services. Other factors, such as better nutrition, sanitation and housing also play a role, particularly in countries with developing economies (OECD, 2004c).

On average across OECD countries, life expectancy at birth for the whole population reached 79.1 years in 2007, a gain of more than ten years since 1960 (Figure 1.1.1). In almost one-half of OECD countries, life expectancy at birth in 2007 exceeded 80 years. The country with the highest life expectancy was Japan, with a life expectancy for women and men combined of 82.6 years. At the other end of the scale, life expectancy in OECD countries was the lowest in Turkey, followed by Hungary. However, while life expectancy in Hungary has increased modestly since 1960, it has increased sharply in Turkey, so that it is rapidly catching up with the OECD average (OECD and the World Bank, 2008). Life expectancy at birth in Korea, Turkey, Ireland and Portugal has increased by three years or more in the ten-year period 1997-2007.

The gender gap in life expectancy stood at 5.6 years on average across OECD countries in 2007, with life expectancy reaching 76.3 years among men and 81.9 years among women (Figure 1.1.2). Between 1960 and 2007, this gender gap widened on average by about half a year. But this result hides different trends between earlier and later decades. While the gender gap in life expectancy increased substantially in many countries during the 1960s and the 1970s, it narrowed during the past 25 years, reflecting higher gains in life expectancy among men than among women in most OECD countries. The recent narrowing of the gender gap in life expectancy can be attributed at least partly to the narrowing of differences in risk-increasing behaviours between men and women, such as smoking, accompanied by sharp reductions in mortality rates from cardio-vascular diseases among men.

Higher national income (as measured by GDP per capita) is generally associated with higher life expectancy at birth, although the relationship is less pronounced at higher levels of national income (Figure 1.1.3). There are also notable differences in life expectancy between OECD countries with similar income per capita. Japan and Spain have higher, and the United States, Denmark and Hungary lower life expectancies than would be predicted by their GDP per capita alone.

Figure 1.1.4 shows the relationship between life expectancy at birth and health expenditure per capita across OECD countries. Higher health spending per capita is generally associated with higher life expectancy at birth, although this relationship tends to be less pronounced in countries with higher health spending per capita. Again, Japan and Spain stand out as having relatively high life expectancies, and the United States, Denmark and Hungary relatively low life expectancies, given their levels of health spending.

Variations in GDP per capita may influence *both* life expectancy and health expenditure per capita. Many other factors, beyond national income and total health spending also explain variations in life expectancy across countries.

Definition and deviations

Life expectancy measures how long on average people would live based on a *given* set of age-specific death rates. However, the *actual* age-specific death rates of any particular birth cohort cannot be known in advance. If age-specific death rates are falling (as has been the case over the past decades in OECD countries), actual life spans will be higher than life expectancy calculated with current death rates.

Each country calculates its life expectancy according to methodologies that can vary somewhat. These differences in methodology can affect the comparability of reported life expectancy estimates, as different methods can change a country's life expectancy estimates by a fraction of a year. Life expectancy at birth for the total population is calculated by the OECD Secretariat for all countries, using the unweighted average of life expectancy of men and women.

1.1.1 Life expectancy at birth, total population, 1960 and 2007 (or latest year available)

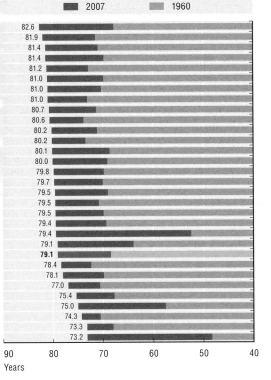

1.1.2 Life expectancy at birth, by gender, 2007 (or latest year available)

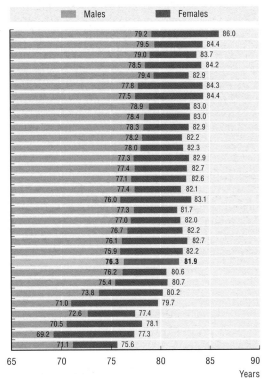

1.1.3 Life expectancy at birth and GDP per capita, 2007 (or latest year available)

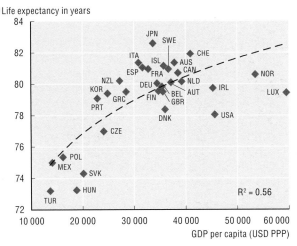

1.1.4 Life expectancy at birth and health spending per capita, 2007 (or latest year available)

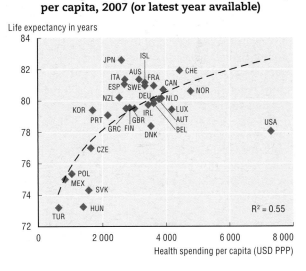

Source: OECD Health Data 2009.

StatLink http://dx.doi.org/10.1787/717383404708

1.2. Life expectancy at age 65

Life expectancy at age 65 has increased significantly among both women and men over the past several decades in all OECD countries. Some of the factors explaining the gains in life expectancy at age 65 include advances in medical care combined with greater access to health care, healthier lifestyles and improved living conditions before and after people reach age 65.

In 2007, life expectancy at age 65 in OECD countries stood, on average, at over 20 years for women and close to 17 years for men (Figure 1.2.1). This represents a gain of almost five years for women and four years for men on average across OECD countries since 1970. Hence, the gender gap in life expectancy at age 65 increased slightly in many countries between 1970 and 2007.

Similarly, life expectancy at age 80 also increased slightly more rapidly among women than among men on average in OECD countries over the past 37 years (Figure 1.2.2). In 2007, life expectancy for women at age 80 stood at 9.2 years (up from 6.5 years in 1970) on average in OECD countries, while the corresponding figure for men was 7.6 years (up from 5.6 years in 1970).

Japan registered particularly strong gains in life expectancy at age 65 in recent decades, with an increase of over eight years for women and six for men between 1970 and 2007. As a result of these large gains, Japanese women and men enjoyed the longest life expectancy at age 65 across all OECD countries in 2007, with respectively 23.6 and 18.6 remaining years of life. These gains in Japan can be explained in part by a marked reduction in death rates from heart disease and cerebro-vascular disease (stroke) among elderly people. Many other OECD countries have also registered significant reductions in mortality from cardio-vascular and cerebro-vascular diseases among elderly populations over the past decades (OECD, 2003a; Moon et al., 2003).

Some countries exhibit different standings when comparing their life expectancies at birth and at age 65. Females in Belgium, the United States and New Zealand improve their position relative to other countries, as do males in the United States, France and Mexico. However, males in the Netherlands, Sweden and Luxembourg, rate lower at 65 years of age, compared with at birth.

Gains in longevity at older ages in recent decades in OECD countries, combined with the trend reduction in fertility rates, are contributing to a steady rise in the proportion of older persons in OECD countries (see Annex Tables A.2 and A.3).

Life expectancy at age 65 is expected to continue to increase in coming decades. Based on the United Nations/World Bank Population Database, life expectancy at age 65 is projected to reach 21.6 years for women and 18.1 years in 2040 for men on average in OECD countries (OECD, 2007d).

Whether longer life expectancy is accompanied by good health and functional status among ageing populations has important implications for health and long-term care systems. Recent OECD work has found that although there is a declining trend in severe disability among elderly populations in some countries (e.g. in the United States, Italy and the Netherlands), this is not universally true (Figure 1.2.3). In some other countries (e.g. in Australia and Canada), the rate of severe disability is stable, and in yet other countries (e.g. in Sweden and Japan) severe limitations in activities of daily living appear to be on the rise over the past five to ten years. Combined with population ageing, these trends suggest that there will be increasing need for long-term care in all OECD countries in coming decades (Lafortune et al., 2007).

Definition and deviations

Life expectancy measures how long on average people at a particular age would live based on current age-specific death rates. However, the *actual* age-specific death rates of any particular birth cohort cannot be known in advance. If age-specific death rates are falling – as has been the case over the past decades in OECD countries – actual life spans will be higher than life expectancy calculated with current death rates.

Countries may calculate life expectancy using methodologies that can vary somewhat. These differences in methodology can affect the comparability of reported life expectancy estimates by a fraction of a year.

1.2.1 Life expectancy at age 65 by gender, 1970 and 2007 (or nearest year available)

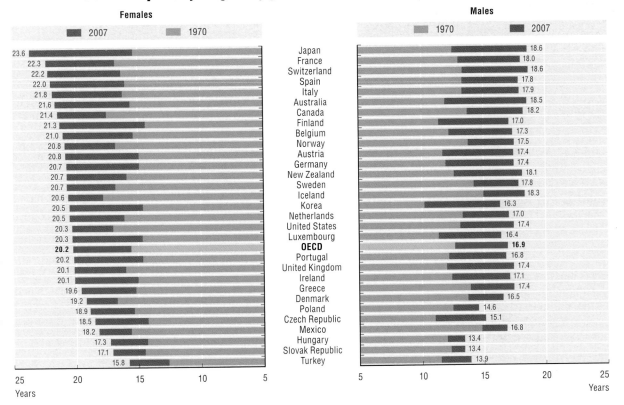

Females

2007 | 1970

Males

1970 | 2007

	Females 2007	Males 2007
Japan	23.6	18.6
France	22.3	18.0
Switzerland	22.2	18.6
Spain	22.0	17.8
Italy	21.8	17.9
Australia	21.6	18.5
Canada	21.4	18.2
Finland	21.3	17.0
Belgium	21.0	17.3
Norway	20.8	17.5
Austria	20.8	17.4
Germany	20.7	17.4
New Zealand	20.7	18.1
Sweden	20.7	17.8
Iceland	20.6	18.3
Korea	20.5	16.3
Netherlands	20.5	17.0
United States	20.3	17.4
Luxembourg	20.3	16.4
OECD	**20.2**	**16.9**
Portugal	20.2	16.8
United Kingdom	20.1	17.4
Ireland	20.1	17.1
Greece	19.6	17.4
Denmark	19.2	16.5
Poland	18.9	14.6
Czech Republic	18.5	15.1
Mexico	18.2	16.8
Hungary	17.3	13.4
Slovak Republic	17.1	13.4
Turkey	15.8	13.9

Years

Years

1.2.2 Trends in life expectancy at age 65 and at age 80, males and females, OECD average, 1970-2007

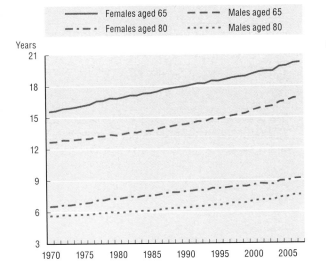

Females aged 65 — — — Males aged 65
— · — · Females aged 80 · · · · · Males aged 80

Years

Source: OECD Health Data 2009.

1.2.3 Trends in severe disability among the population aged 65 and over, selected OECD countries, 1980-2005

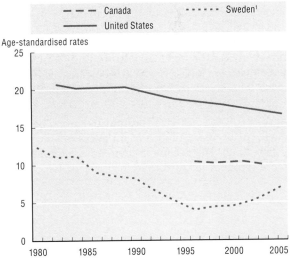

— — — Canada · · · · · · Sweden[1]
——— United States

Age-standardised rates

1. For Sweden, the data relate only to the population aged 65-84.

Source: Lafortune et al. (2007).

StatLink ⬛📊 http://dx.doi.org/10.1787/717451135213

1.3. Premature mortality

Premature mortality, measured in terms of potential years of life lost (PYLL) before the age of 70 years, focuses on deaths among younger age groups of the population. PYLL values are heavily influenced by infant mortality and deaths from diseases and injuries affecting children and younger adults: a death at five years of age represents 65 PYLL; one at 60 years of age only ten. Declines in PYLL can be influenced by advances in medical technology, for example, in relation to infant mortality and deaths due to heart disease, and in prevention and control measures, reducing untimely or avoidable deaths from injuries and communicable diseases. A number of other variables, such as GDP per capita, occupational status, numbers of doctors and alcohol and tobacco consumption, have also been associated with reduced premature mortality (Or, 2000; Joumard et al., 2008).

Rates of premature mortality are higher among males in all countries, with the OECD average in 2006 (4 853 years lost per 100 000 males) almost twice that of females (2 548). The main causes of potential years of life lost before age 70 among men are external causes including accidents and violence (29%), followed by cancer (20%) and circulatory diseases (16%). For women, the principal causes are cancer (31%), external causes (17%), and circulatory diseases (12%).

Among males, Sweden and Iceland had the lowest levels of premature mortality in 2006, and for females levels were lowest in Japan and Italy (Figure 1.3.1). Mexico and Hungary reported the highest premature mortality rates for both males and females, with levels more than double those of the lowest OECD country. The rate for the United States was also high – 30% above the OECD average in the case of males, and 43% for females. Among US males, one-third (and in females, one-fifth) of these premature mortality rates can be attributed to deaths resulting from external causes, including accidents, suicides and homicides. Premature death from homicides for men in the United States is over five times the OECD average.

Across OECD countries, premature mortality has been cut by more than half on average since 1970 (Figure 1.3.2). The decline in premature mortality was more rapid for females than for males between 1970

and the early 1990s, but since then the average rate of PYLL has been declining at the same rate for men and women. The downward trend in infant mortality has been a major factor contributing to the decline in earlier years (see Indicator 1.8 "Infant mortality"). More recently, the decline in deaths from heart disease among adults has contributed significantly to the overall reduction in premature mortality in many countries (see Indicator 1.4 "Mortality from heart disease and stroke").

Portugal and Italy have seen premature mortality rates decline rapidly among both males and females to stand currently at less than one-third of 1970 levels. Although levels are still high, Mexico has also seen a dramatic decline. In each case, the sharp reduction in infant mortality rates has been an important contributing factor. In contrast, premature mortality has declined more slowly in Hungary, particularly among males. This is largely attributed to persistently high levels of mortality from circulatory disease (currently twice the OECD average) and from liver disease (over three times the OECD average). These reflect unhealthy lifestyles, in particular alcohol and tobacco consumption among males in Hungary, together with high suicide rates. Declines in premature mortality have also been slow in Poland and the United States.

Definition and deviations

Potential years of life lost (PYLL) is a summary measure of premature mortality providing an explicit way of weighting deaths occurring at younger ages. The calculation for PYLL involves adding age-specific deaths occurring at each age and weighing them by the number of remaining years to live up to a selected age limit, defined here as age 70. For example, a death occurring at five years of age is counted as 65 years of PYLL. The indicator is expressed per 100 000 females and males.

1.3.1 Potential years of life lost (PYLL), females and males, 2006 (or latest year available)

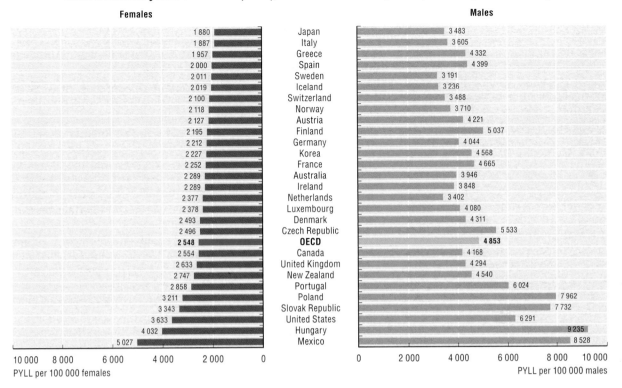

Females — PYLL per 100 000 females

Country	Females	Males
Japan	1 880	3 483
Italy	1 887	3 605
Greece	1 957	4 332
Spain	2 000	4 399
Sweden	2 011	3 191
Iceland	2 019	3 236
Switzerland	2 100	3 488
Norway	2 118	3 710
Austria	2 127	4 221
Finland	2 195	5 037
Germany	2 212	4 044
Korea	2 227	4 568
France	2 252	4 665
Australia	2 289	3 946
Ireland	2 289	3 848
Netherlands	2 377	3 402
Luxembourg	2 378	4 080
Denmark	2 493	4 311
Czech Republic	2 496	5 533
OECD	**2 548**	**4 853**
Canada	2 554	4 168
United Kingdom	2 633	4 294
New Zealand	2 747	4 540
Portugal	2 858	6 024
Poland	3 211	7 962
Slovak Republic	3 343	7 732
United States	3 633	6 291
Hungary	4 032	9 235
Mexico	5 027	8 528

Males — PYLL per 100 000 males

1.3.2 Reduction in potential years of life lost (PYLL), females and males combined, 1970-2006 (or nearest year)

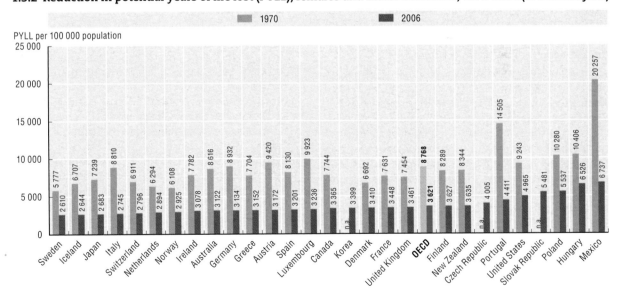

PYLL per 100 000 population

	1970	2006
Sweden	5 777	2 610
Iceland	6 707	2 644
Japan	7 239	2 683
Italy	8 810	2 745
Switzerland	6 911	2 796
Netherlands	6 294	2 894
Norway	6 108	2 925
Ireland	7 782	3 078
Australia	8 616	3 122
Germany	8 932	3 134
Greece	7 704	3 152
Austria	9 420	3 172
Spain	8 130	3 201
Luxembourg	9 923	3 236
Canada	7 744	3 365
Korea	n.a.	3 399
Denmark	6 692	3 410
France	7 631	3 448
United Kingdom	7 454	3 461
OECD	**8 768**	**3 621**
Finland	8 289	3 627
New Zealand	8 344	3 635
Czech Republic	n.a.	4 005
Portugal	14 505	4 411
United States	9 243	4 965
Slovak Republic	n.a.	5 481
Poland	10 280	5 537
Hungary	10 406	6 526
Mexico	20 257	6 737

Source: OECD Health Data 2009. The raw mortality data are extracted from the WHO Mortality Database.

StatLink 🖳 http://dx.doi.org/10.1787/717458111254

1.4. Mortality from heart disease and stroke

Cardiovascular diseases are the main cause of mortality in almost all OECD countries, accounting for 36% of all deaths in 2006. They cover a range of diseases related to the circulatory system, including ischemic heart disease (known as IHD, or heart attack) and cerebro-vascular disease (or stroke). Together, IHD and stroke comprise two-thirds of all cardiovascular deaths, and caused one-quarter of all deaths in OECD countries in 2006.

Ischemic heart disease is caused by the accumulation of fatty deposits lining the inner wall of a coronary artery, restricting blood flow to the heart. IHD alone was responsible for 16% of all deaths in OECD countries in 2006. Mortality from IHD varies considerably, however, across OECD countries (Figure 1.4.1). Central and eastern European countries report the highest IHD mortality rates, the Slovak Republic for both males and females, followed by Hungary and the Czech Republic. IHD mortality rates are also relatively high in Finland, Poland and the United States, with rates several times higher than in Japan and Korea. There are regional patterns to the variability in IHD mortality rates. Closely following the two OECD Asian countries, the countries with the lowest IHD mortality rates are four countries located in southern Europe: France, Spain, Portugal and Italy. This lends support to the commonly held hypothesis that there are underlying risk factors, such as diet, which explain differences in IHD mortality across countries.

Death rates are much higher for men than for women in all countries (Figure 1.4.1). On average across OECD countries, IHD mortality rates in 2006 were nearly two times greater for men than for women.

Since 1980, IHD mortality rates have declined in nearly all OECD countries. The decline has been most remarkable in Denmark, the Netherlands, Sweden, Norway and Australia, with IHD mortality rates being cut by two-thirds or more. A number of factors are responsible, with declining tobacco consumption contributing to reducing the incidence of IHD, and consequently reducing IHD mortality rates. Significant improvements in medical care for treating IHD have also contributed to reducing mortality rates (Moïse et al., 2003) (see Indicators 4.6 "Cardiac proce-

dures" and 5.4 "In-hospital mortality following acute myocardial infarction"). A small number of countries, however, have seen little or no decline since 1980. In Hungary and Poland, mortality rates have increased. The rate in Greece has declined only slightly, although it was already comparatively low in 1980.

Stroke is another important cause of mortality in OECD countries, accounting for about 9% of all deaths in 2006. It is caused by the disruption of the blood supply to the brain, and in addition to being an important cause of mortality, the disability burden from stroke is substantial (Moon et al., 2003). As with IHD, there are large variations in stroke mortality rates across countries (Figure 1.4.1). The rates are highest in Portugal, Hungary, the Czech Republic and Greece. They are the lowest in Switzerland, France, Canada and the United States.

Looking at trends over time, stroke mortality has decreased in all OECD countries (except Poland) since 1980. Rates have declined by almost three-quarters in Austria, Japan, Luxembourg, Ireland and France. As with IHD, the reduction in stroke mortality can be attributed at least partly to a reduction in risk factors. Tobacco smoking and hypertension are the main modifiable risk factors for stroke. Improvements in medical treatment for stroke have also increased survival rates (see Indicator 5.5 "In-hospital mortality following stroke").

Definition and deviations

Mortality rates are based on the crude number of deaths according to selected causes in the WHO Mortality Database. Mathers et al. (2005) have provided a general assessment of the coverage, completeness and reliability of WHO data on causes of death. Mortality rates have been age-standardised to the 1980 OECD population, to remove variations arising from differences in age structures across countries and over time within each country.

1.4.1 Ischemic heart disease, mortality rates, 2006 (or latest year available)

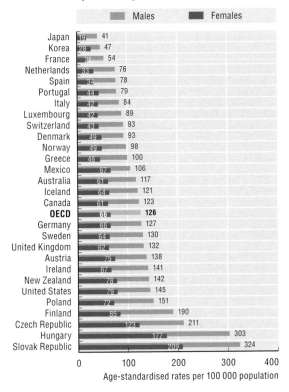

Age-standardised rates per 100 000 population

1.4.2 Stroke, mortality rates, 2006 (or latest year available)

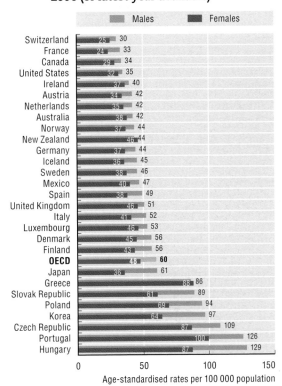

Age-standardised rates per 100 000 population

1.4.3 Trends in ischemic heart disease mortality rates, selected OECD countries, 1980-2006

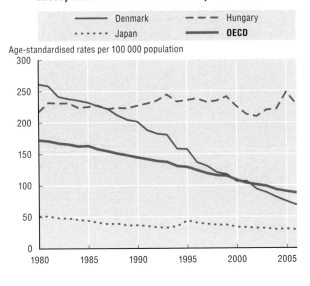

1.4.4 Trends in stroke mortality rates, selected OECD countries, 1980-2006

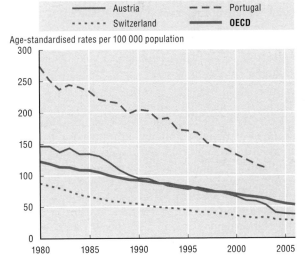

Source: OECD Health Data 2009. The raw mortality data are extracted from the WHO Mortality Database, and age-standardised to the 1980 OECD population.

StatLink ⟶ http://dx.doi.org/10.1787/717474000840

1.5. Mortality from cancer

Cancer is the second leading cause of mortality in OECD countries (after diseases of the circulatory system), accounting for 27% of all deaths on average in 2006. In 2006, cancer mortality rates were the lowest in Mexico, Finland, Switzerland and Japan. They were the highest in central and eastern European countries (Hungary, the Czech and Slovak Republics, Poland) and Denmark (Figure 1.5.1).

Cancer mortality rates are higher for men than for women in all OECD countries (Figure 1.5.1). In 2006, the gender gap in death rates from cancer was particularly wide in Korea, Spain, the Slovak Republic, Japan and France, with mortality rates among men more than twice as high as for women. The gender gap in cancer mortality rates can be explained partly by the greater prevalence of risk factors among men, as well as the lesser availability or use of screening programmes for different types of cancers affecting men, leading to lower survival rates after diagnosis.

Lung cancer still accounts for the greatest number of cancer deaths among men in all OECD countries (except Mexico and Sweden), while it is also one of the main causes of cancer mortality among women. Tobacco smoking is the most important risk factor for lung cancer. In 2006, death rates from lung cancer among men were the highest in central and eastern European countries (Hungary, Poland, the Slovak and Czech Republics), the Netherlands, Greece and Korea (Figure 1.5.2). These are all countries where smoking rates among men are relatively high. Death rates from lung cancer among men are low in Mexico, and in Sweden, one of the countries with the lowest smoking rate among men (see Indicator 2.5 "Tobacco consumption").

Breast cancer is the most common form of cancer among women in all OECD countries (IARC, 2004). It accounts for 30% or more of cancer incidence among women, and 15% to 20% of cancer deaths. While there has been an increase in measured incidence rates of breast cancer over the past decade, death rates have declined or remained stable, indicating increases in survival rates due to earlier diagnosis and/or better treatments (see Indicator 5.8 "Screening, survival and mortality for breast cancer"). The lowest mortality rates from breast cancer are in Korea and Japan, while the highest mortality rates are in Denmark, the Netherlands, Ireland and the United Kingdom (Figure 1.5.3).

Prostate cancer has become the most commonly occurring cancer among men in many OECD countries, particularly for those aged over 65 years of age, although death rates from prostate cancer remain lower than for lung cancer in all countries except Mexico and Sweden. The rise in the reported incidence of prostate cancer in many countries during the 1990s and 2000s is largely due to the greater use of prostate-specific antigen (PSA) diagnostic tests. Death rates from prostate cancer in 2006 varied from lows of less than 10 per 100 000 males in Korea and Japan, to highs of more than 30 per 100 000 males in Denmark, Sweden and Norway (Figure 1.5.4). The causes of prostate cancer are not well-understood. Some evidence suggests that environmental and dietary factors might influence the risk of prostate cancer (Institute of Cancer Research, 2009).

Death rates from all types of cancer for males and females have declined at least slightly in most OECD countries since 1985, although the decline has been more modest than for cardio-vascular diseases, explaining why cancer accounts now for a larger share of all deaths. The exceptions to this declining pattern are Greece, Korea, Poland, Portugal, the Slovak Republic and Spain, where cancer mortality has remained static or increased between 1985 and 2006.

Definition and deviations

Mortality rates are based on the crude number of deaths according to selected causes in the WHO Mortality Database. Mathers *et al.* (2005) have provided a general assessment of the coverage, completeness and reliability of WHO data on causes of death. The international comparability of cancer mortality data can be affected by differences in medical training and practices as well as in death certification procedures across countries. Mortality rates have been age-standardised to the 1980 OECD population, to remove variations arising from differences in age structures across countries and over time within each country.

1.5.1 All cancers, mortality rates, males and females, 2006 (or latest year available)

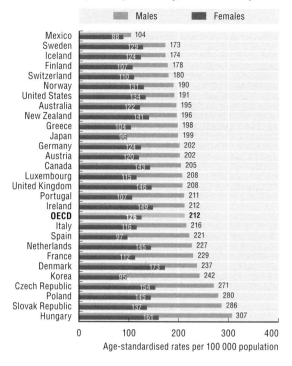

1.5.2 Lung cancers, mortality rates, males and females, 2006 (or latest year available)

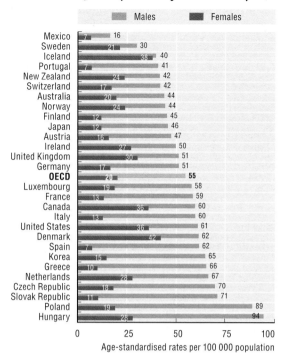

1.5.3 Breast cancers, mortality rates, females, 2006 (or latest year available)

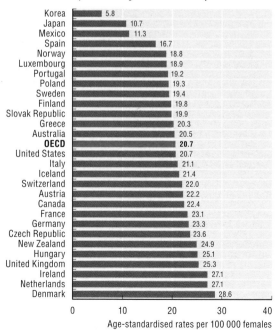

1.5.4 Prostate cancers, mortality rates, males, 2006 (or latest year available)

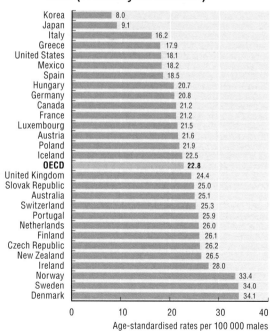

Source: OECD Health Data 2009. The raw mortality data are extracted from the WHO Mortality Database, and age-standardised to the 1980 OECD population.

StatLink ᝲᝲᎦᎦ http://dx.doi.org/10.1787/717484673283

1.6. Mortality from road accidents

Worldwide, an estimated 1.2 million people are killed in road traffic accidents each year, and as many as 50 million people are injured or disabled (WHO, 2009c). In OECD countries alone, they were responsible for more than 125 000 deaths in 2006, occurring most often in the United States (46 000), Mexico (17 000) and Japan (9 000). Around 5 000-6 000 road accident deaths occurred in each of Italy, Poland and Germany in 2006.

Mortality from road accidents is the leading cause of death among children and young people, and especially young men, in many countries. The fatality risk for motor cycles and mopeds is highest among all modes of transport, even though most fatal traffic injuries occur in passenger vehicles (ETSC, 2003; Beck et al., 2007).

Besides the adverse social, physical and psychological effects, the direct and indirect financial costs of road traffic accidents are substantial; one estimate put these at 2% of gross national product annually in highly-motorised countries (Peden et al., 2004). Injury and mortality from road accidents remains a serious public health concern.

Death rates were the highest in 2006 in Mexico and Portugal, followed by Korea and the United States, all in excess of 15 deaths per 100 000 population (Figure 1.6.1). They were the lowest in the Netherlands, Norway and Sweden, at five deaths per 100 000 population or less. A four-fold difference exists between the Netherlands and Mexico, the countries with the lowest and highest rates. Deaths from road accidents are much higher for males than for females in all OECD countries, with disparities in rates ranging from twice as high among males in Iceland to more than four times higher in Greece and Italy. On average, three times as many males than females die in road accidents (Figure 1.6.2).

Much road accident injury and mortality is preventable. Road security has increased greatly over the past decades in many countries through improvements of road systems, education and prevention campaigns, the adoption of new laws and regulations and the enforcement of these new laws through more traffic controls. As a result, death rates due to road accidents have been cut by more than half on average in OECD countries since 1970 (Figure 1.6.3). The Netherlands, Germany and Switzerland have seen the largest declines in death rates, with a reduction of about 80% since 1970, although vehicle kilometers travelled have increased by 2.7 times on average in European countries in the same period (OECD/ITF, 2008). Death rates have also declined in the United States, but at a slower pace, and therefore remain above the OECD average. In Mexico and Greece, there have been significant increases in death rates from road accidents since 1970 (Figure 1.6.4).

Based on an extrapolation of past trends, projections from the World Bank indicate that between 2000 and 2020, road traffic deaths may decline further by about 30% in high-income countries, but may increase substantially in low- and middle-income countries if no additional road safety counter-measures are put in place (Peden et al., 2004).

Definition and deviations

Mortality rates are based on the crude number of deaths according to selected causes in the WHO Mortality Database. Mathers et al. (2005) have provided a general assessment of the coverage, completeness and reliability of WHO data on causes of death. Mortality rates have been age-standardised to the 1980 OECD population, to remove variations arising from differences in age structures across countries and over time within each country.

Mortality rates from road traffic accidents in Luxembourg are biased upward because of the large volume of traffic in transit, resulting in a significant proportion of non-residents killed.

1.6.1 Road accidents, mortality rates, total population, 2006 (or latest year available)

1.6.2 Road accidents, mortality rates, males and females, 2006 (or latest year available)

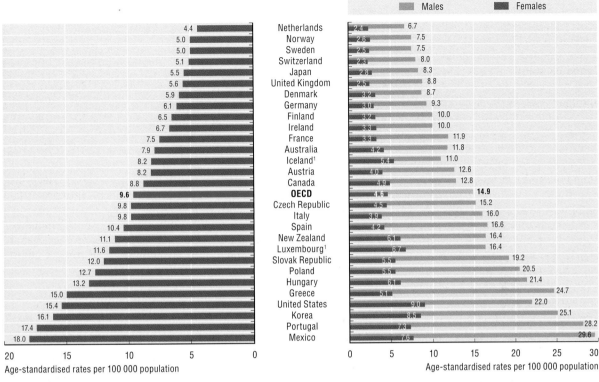

Age-standardised rates per 100 000 population

1. Three-year average.

1.6.3 Trends in road accident mortality rates, selected OECD countries, 1970-2006

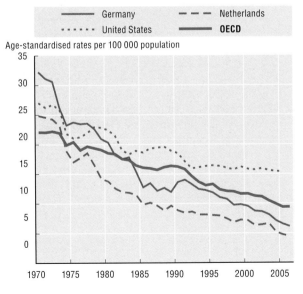

1.6.4 Change in road accident mortality rates, 1970-2006 (or nearest year)

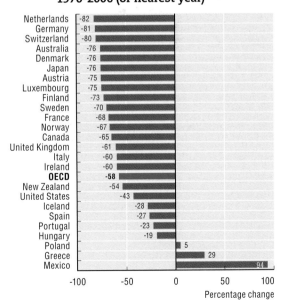

Source: OECD Health Data 2009. The raw mortality data have been extracted from the WHO Mortality Database, and age-standardised to the 1980 OECD population.

StatLink ᐧᒪᔕᐧ http://dx.doi.org/10.1787/717527613871

The intentional killing of oneself is evidence not only of personal breakdown, but also of a deterioration of the social context in which an individual lives. Suicide may be the end-point of a number of different contributing factors. It is more likely to occur during crisis periods associated with divorce, alcohol and drug abuse, unemployment, clinical depression and other forms of mental illness. Because of this, suicide is often used as a proxy indicator of the mental health status of a population. However, the number of suicides in certain countries may be under-estimated because of the stigma that is associated with the act, or because of data issues associated with reporting criteria (see "Definition and deviations").

Suicide is a significant cause of death in many OECD countries, and there were 140 000 such deaths in 2006. In 2006, there were fewest suicides in southern European countries (Greece, Italy and Spain) and in Mexico and the United Kingdom, at less than seven deaths per 100 000 population (Figure 1.7.1). They were highest in Korea, Hungary, Japan and Finland, at 18 or more deaths per 100 000 population. There is more than a seven-fold difference between Korea and Greece, the countries with the lowest and high death rates.

Since 1990, suicide rates have decreased in many OECD countries, with pronounced declines of 40% or more in Denmark, Luxembourg and Hungary (Figure 1.7.3). Despite this progress, Hungary still has one of the highest rates among OECD countries. On the other hand, death rates from suicides have increased the most since 1990 in Korea, Mexico and Japan, although in Mexico rates remain at low levels. In Korea and Japan, suicide rates now stand well above the OECD average (Figure 1.7.4). Male suicide rates in Korea almost tripled from 12 per 100 000 in 1990 to 32 in 2006, and suicide rates among women are the highest among OECD countries, at 13 per 100 000. Economic downturn, weakening social integration and the erosion of the traditional family support base for the elderly have all been implicated in Korea's recent increase in suicide rates (Kwon et al., 2009).

In general, death rates from suicides are three to four times greater for men than for women across OECD countries (Figure 1.7.2), and this gender gap has been fairly stable over time. The gender gap is narrower for attempted suicides, reflecting the fact that women tend to use less fatal methods than men.

Suicide is also related to age, with young people aged under 25 and elderly people especially at risk. While suicide rates among the latter have generally declined over the past two decades, almost no progress has been observed among younger people.

Since suicides are, in the vast majority of cases, linked with depression and alcohol and other substance abuse, the early detection of these psycho-social problems in high-risk groups by families, social workers and health professionals must be part of suicide prevention campaigns, together with the provision of effective support and treatment. With suicide receiving increasing attention worldwide, many countries are promoting mental health and developing national strategies for prevention, focussing on at-risk groups (Hawton and van Heeringen, 2009). In Finland and Iceland, suicide prevention programmes have been based on efforts to promote strong multisectoral collaboration and networking (NOMESCO, 2007).

Definition and deviations

The World Health Organisation defines "suicide" as an act deliberately initiated and performed by a person in the full knowledge or expectation of its fatal outcome.

Mortality rates are based on the crude number of deaths according to selected causes in the WHO Mortality Database. Mathers et al. (2005) have provided a general assessment of the coverage, completeness and reliability of WHO data on causes of death. Mortality rates have been age-standardised to the 1980 OECD population, to remove variations arising from differences in age structures across countries and over time within each country.

Comparability of suicide data between countries is affected by a number of reporting criteria, including how a person's intention of killing themselves is ascertained, who is responsible for completing the death certificate, whether a forensic investigation is carried out, and the provisions for confidentiality of the cause of death. Caution is required therefore in interpreting variations across countries.

1.7.1 Suicide, mortality rates, total population, 2006 (or latest year available)

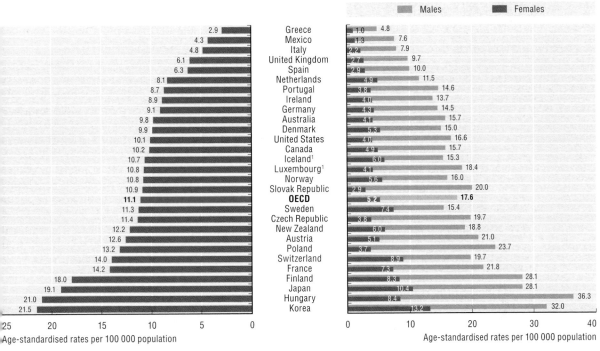

Country	Rate
Greece	2.9
Mexico	4.3
Italy	4.8
United Kingdom	6.1
Spain	6.3
Netherlands	8.1
Portugal	8.7
Ireland	8.9
Germany	9.1
Australia	9.8
Denmark	9.9
United States	10.1
Canada	10.2
Iceland[1]	10.7
Luxembourg[1]	10.8
Norway	10.8
Slovak Republic	10.9
OECD	**11.1**
Sweden	11.3
Czech Republic	11.4
New Zealand	12.2
Austria	12.6
Poland	13.2
Switzerland	14.0
France	14.2
Finland	18.0
Japan	19.1
Hungary	21.0
Korea	21.5

Age-standardised rates per 100 000 population

1. Three-year average.

1.7.2 Suicide, mortality rates, males and females, 2006 (or latest year available)

Country	Females	Males
Greece	1.0	4.8
Mexico	1.3	7.6
Italy	2.2	7.9
United Kingdom	2.7	9.7
Spain	2.9	10.0
Netherlands	4.9	11.5
Portugal	3.8	14.6
Ireland	4.0	13.7
Germany	4.3	14.5
Australia	4.1	15.7
Denmark	5.3	15.0
United States	4.0	16.6
Canada	4.9	15.7
Iceland[1]	6.0	15.3
Luxembourg[1]	4.1	18.4
Norway	5.6	16.0
Slovak Republic	2.9	20.0
OECD	**5.2**	**17.6**
Sweden	7.4	15.4
Czech Republic	3.8	19.7
New Zealand	6.0	18.8
Austria	5.1	21.0
Poland	3.7	23.7
Switzerland	8.9	19.7
France	7.3	21.8
Finland	8.3	28.1
Japan	10.4	28.1
Hungary	8.4	36.3
Korea	13.2	32.0

Age-standardised rates per 100 000 population

1.7.3 Change in suicide rates, 1990-2006 (or nearest year)

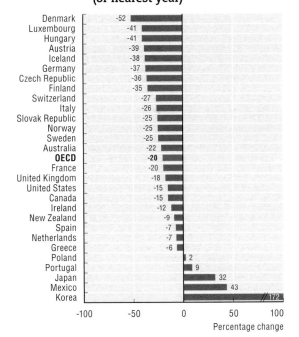

Country	Percentage change
Denmark	-52
Luxembourg	-41
Hungary	-41
Austria	-39
Iceland	-38
Germany	-37
Czech Republic	-36
Finland	-35
Switzerland	-27
Italy	-26
Slovak Republic	-25
Norway	-25
Sweden	-25
Australia	-22
OECD	**-20**
France	-20
United Kingdom	-18
United States	-15
Canada	-15
Ireland	-12
New Zealand	-9
Spain	-7
Netherlands	-7
Greece	-6
Poland	2
Portugal	9
Japan	32
Mexico	43
Korea	172

Percentage change

1.7.4 Trends in suicide rates, selected OECD countries, 1990-2006

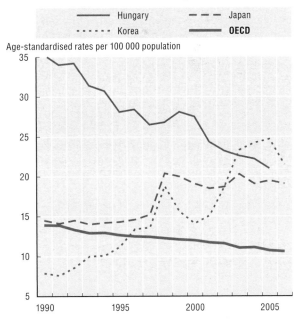

Age-standardised rates per 100 000 population

Legend: Hungary — ; Japan – – –; Korea ·······; OECD ——

Source: OECD Health Data 2009. The raw mortality data have been extracted from the WHO Mortality Database, and age-standardised to the 1980 OECD population.

StatLink http://dx.doi.org/10.1787/717546558510

Infant mortality, the rate at which babies of less than one year of age die, reflects the effect of economic and social conditions on the health of mothers and new-borns as well as the effectiveness of health systems.

In 2007, infant mortality rates in OECD countries ranged from a low of two to three deaths per 1 000 live births in Japan, Nordic countries (with the exception of Denmark), Ireland and Luxembourg, up to a high of 16 and 21 deaths per 1 000 live births in Mexico and Turkey respectively (Figure 1.8.1). Infant mortality rates were also relatively high (six or more deaths per 1 000 live births) in the United States and in some eastern and central European countries. Excluding Turkey and Mexico, the average across the remaining 28 OECD countries was 3.9 in 2007.

Around two-thirds of the deaths that occur during the first year of life are neonatal deaths (i.e. during the first four weeks). Birth defects, prematurity and other conditions arising during pregnancy are the principal factors contributing to neonatal mortality in developed countries. With an increasing number of women deferring childbearing and the rise in multiple births linked with fertility treatments, the number of pre-term births has tended to increase (see Indicator 1.9 "Infant health: low birth weight"). In a number of higher-income countries, this has contributed to a leveling-off of the downward trend in infant mortality rates over the past few years. The increase in the birth of very small infants was the main reason for the first increase since the 1950s in infant mortality rates in the United States between 2001 and 2002. For deaths beyond a month (post neonatal mortality), there tends to be a greater range of causes – the most common being SIDS (Sudden Infant Death Syndrome), birth defects, infections and accidents.

All OECD countries have achieved remarkable progress in reducing infant mortality rates from the levels of 1970, when the average was approaching 30 deaths per 1 000 live births (Figure 1.8.3). This equates to a cumulative reduction of over 80% since 1970. Portugal has seen its infant mortality rate reduced by more than 7% per year on average since 1970, going from the country with the highest rate in Europe to an infant mortality rate among the lowest in the OECD in 2007 (Figure 1.8.2). Large reductions in infant mortality rates have also been observed in Korea and Luxembourg. On the other hand, the reduction in infant mortality rates has been slower in the Netherlands and the United States. Infant mortality rates in the United States used to be well below the OECD average (and median), but they are now above average (Figure 1.8.3).

Numerous studies have used infant mortality rates as a health outcome to examine the effect of a variety of medical and non-medical determinants of health (e.g. Joumard et al., 2008). Although most analyses show an overall negative relationship between infant mortality and health spending, the fact that some countries with a high level of health expenditure do not necessarily exhibit low levels of infant mortality has led some researchers to conclude that more health spending is not necessarily required to obtain better results (Retzlaff-Roberts et al., 2004). A body of research also suggests that many factors beyond the quality and efficiency of the health system, such as income inequality, the social environment, and individual lifestyles and attitudes, influence infant mortality rates (Kiely et al., 1995).

Definition and deviations

The infant mortality rate is the number of deaths of children under one year of age in a given year, expressed per 1 000 live births. Neonatal mortality refers to the death of children under 28 days.

Some of the international variation in infant and neonatal mortality rates may be due to variations among countries in registering practices of premature infants. Most countries have no gestational age or weight limits for mortality registration. Minimal limits exist for Norway (to be counted as a death following a live birth, the gestational age must exceed 12 weeks) and in the Czech Republic, France, the Netherlands and Poland a minimum gestational age of 22 weeks and/or a weight threshold of 500 g is applied.

1.8.1 Infant mortality rates, 2007 (or latest year available)

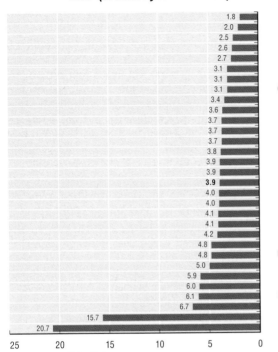

	Deaths per 1 000 live births
Luxembourg	1.8
Iceland	2.0
Sweden	2.5
Japan	2.6
Finland	2.7
Ireland	3.1
Norway	3.1
Czech Republic	3.1
Portugal	3.4
Greece	3.6
Austria	3.7
Italy	3.7
Spain	3.7
France	3.8
Germany	3.9
Switzerland	3.9
OECD[1]	**3.9**
Belgium	4.0
Denmark	4.0
Korea	4.1
Netherlands	4.1
Australia	4.2
New Zealand	4.8
United Kingdom	4.8
Canada	5.0
Hungary	5.9
Poland	6.0
Slovak Republic	6.1
United States	6.7
Mexico	15.7
Turkey	20.7

1.8.2 Decline in infant mortality rates, 1970-2007 (or nearest year)

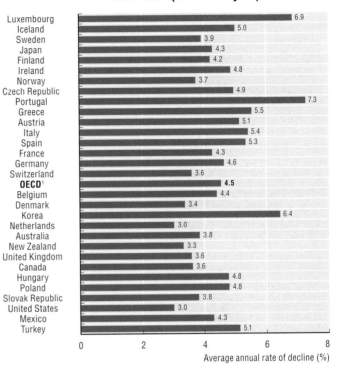

	Average annual rate of decline (%)
Luxembourg	6.9
Iceland	5.0
Sweden	3.9
Japan	4.3
Finland	4.2
Ireland	4.8
Norway	3.7
Czech Republic	4.9
Portugal	7.3
Greece	5.5
Austria	5.1
Italy	5.4
Spain	5.3
France	4.3
Germany	4.6
Switzerland	3.6
OECD[1]	**4.5**
Belgium	4.4
Denmark	3.4
Korea	6.4
Netherlands	3.0
Australia	3.8
New Zealand	3.3
United Kingdom	3.6
Canada	3.6
Hungary	4.8
Poland	4.8
Slovak Republic	3.8
United States	3.0
Mexico	4.3
Turkey	5.1

1. Because of their high rates, Mexico and Turkey are excluded from the OECD average.

1.8.3 Infant mortality rates, selected OECD countries, 1970-2007

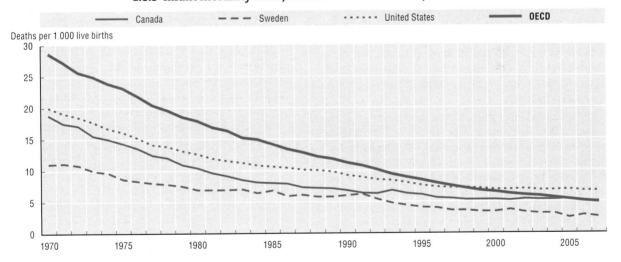

Source: OECD Health Data 2009.

StatLink ⚌ http://dx.doi.org/10.1787/717581042734

1.9. Infant health: low birth weight

Low birth weight – defined here as newborns weighing less than 2 500 grams – is an important indicator of infant health because of the close relationship between birth weight and infant morbidity and mortality. There are two categories of low birth weight babies: those occurring as a result of restricted foetal growth and those resulting from pre-term birth. Low birth weight infants have a greater risk of poor health or death, require a longer period of hospitalisation after birth, and are more likely to develop significant disabilities (UNICEF and WHO, 2004). Risk factors for low birth weight include being an adolescent mother, having a previous history of low weight births, harmful behaviours such as smoking, excessive alcohol consumption and poor nutrition, a low Body Mass Index, a background of low parental socio-economic status or minority race, as well as having in-vitro fertilisation treatment (IHE, 2008).

In 2007, the Nordic countries – including Iceland, Sweden and Finland – reported the smallest proportions of low weight births, with less than 4.5% of live births defined as low birth weight. Turkey, Japan, Greece, the United States and Hungary are at the other end of the scale, with rates of low birth weight infants above 8% (Figure 1.9.1). These figures compare with an overall OECD average of 6.8%.

Since 1980 the prevalence of low birth weight infants has increased in a number of OECD countries (Figure 1.9.2). There may be several reasons for this rise. First, the number of multiple births, with the increased risks of pre-term births and low birth weight, has risen steadily, partly as a result of the rise in fertility treatments. Other factors which may have influenced the rise in low birth weight are older age at childbearing and increases in the use of delivery management techniques such as induction of labour and caesarean delivery.

Japan, Portugal and Spain, historically among a group of countries with a low proportion of low birth weight, have seen great increases in the past 25 years. As a result, the proportion of low birth weight babies in these countries is now above the OECD average (Figure 1.9.3). In the case of Japan, a number of risk factors have been cited as contributing to this increase, including the rising prevalence in smoking among younger women from the 1970s onwards together with a significant move towards later

motherhood (Ohmi et al., 2001). Despite the increase in low birth weight babies, Japanese medical care for newborns has been particularly successful in reducing infant mortality.

Figure 1.9.4 shows some correlation between the percentage of low birth weight infants and infant mortality rates. In general, countries reporting a low proportion of low birth weight infants also report relatively low infant mortality rates. This is the case for instance for the Nordic countries. Japan, however, is an exception, reporting the highest proportion of low birth weight infants but one of the lowest infant mortality rates.

Comparisons of different population groups within countries show that the proportion of low birth weight infants is also be influenced by differences in education, income and associated living conditions. In the United States, marked differences between groups in the proportion of low birth weight infants have been observed, with black infants having a rate almost double that of white infants (CDC, 2009a). Similar differences have also been observed among the indigenous and non-indigenous populations in Australia (Laws and Hilder, 2008) and Mexico, reflecting the disadvantaged living conditions of many of these mothers.

Definition and deviations

Low birth weight is defined by the World Health Organisation (WHO) as the weight of an infant at birth of less than 2 500 grams (5.5 pounds) irrespective of the gestational age of the infant. This is based on epidemiological observations regarding the increased risk of death to the infant and serves for international comparative health statistics. The number of low weight births is then expressed as a percentage of total live births.

The majority of the data comes from birth registers, however for Mexico the source is a national health interview survey. A small number of countries supply data for selected regions or hospital sectors only.

1.9.1 Low birth weight infants, 2007 (or latest year available)

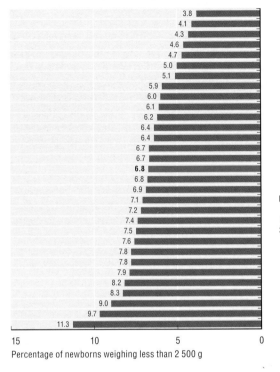

Percentage of newborns weighing less than 2 500 g

1.9.2 Change in proportion of low birth weight infants, 1980-2007

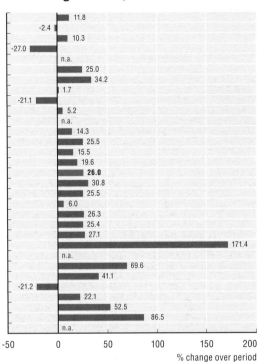

% change over period

1.9.3 Trends in low birth weight infants, selected OECD countries, 1980-2007

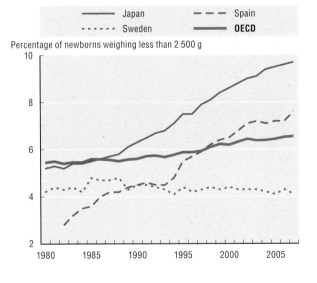

1.9.4 Low birth weight and infant mortality, 2007 (or latest year available)

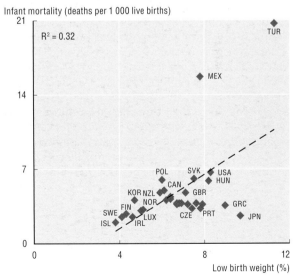

Source: OECD Health Data 2009.

StatLink http://dx.doi.org/10.1787/717583038273

1.10. Dental health among children

Dental problems, mostly in the form of caries (tooth decay) and gum disease, are common in developed countries, affecting 60-90% of school children and the vast majority of adults (WHO, 2003). People with poor oral health may experience pain and discomfort, functional impairment, low self-esteem and dissatisfaction with their appearance. Dental and other oral diseases thus represent a major public health problem. Dental diseases are highly related to lifestyle factors, which include a high sugar diet, while also reflecting whether or not protective measures such as exposure to fluoride and good oral hygiene are present. Much of the burden of dental disease falls on disadvantaged and socially marginalised populations (WHO, 2003), and children are especially vulnerable. Treatment of dental disease in developed countries is often costly, although many countries offer free or subsidised dental care for children and adolescents (see also Indicator 6.6 "Inequalities in dentist consultations").

In 2006, or the closest available year, 12-year-old children in Germany, the United Kingdom, Denmark, Luxembourg, the Netherlands and Switzerland had an average of less than one decayed, missing or filled permanent tooth (DMFT) (Figure 1.10.1). In contrast, children in Poland and Hungary had a DMFT score of three or more. Most OECD countries had a very low to low score of between one and two DMFT for 12-year-old children.

The past 25 years have seen substantial falls in the DMFT index across OECD countries, declining from an average 4.7 in 1980, to 2.7 in 1990, and 1.5 in 2006 for a consistent group of countries with long time series (Figure 1.10.3). During that period, all but one country (Poland) for which data are available saw declines in DMFT of 50% or more (Figure 1.10.2) – a substantial public health achievement. Almost all OECD countries were able to meet the World Health Organisation target of no more than three DMFT by the year 2000 (WHO, 2003). However, there is cause for concern among some countries such as Australia, Austria and the United States, which have seen a slowing of the decline, or even an increase in DMFT in recent years.

Reductions in caries and other dental problems were achieved through numerous public health measures such as community water fluoridation, along with changing living conditions, disease management and improving oral hygiene. Dentistry and oral health is moving towards preventive and minimally invasive care, meaning that national strategies are being integrated with broader chronic disease prevention and general health promotion goals, since the risks for each are linked (European Commission, 2008b; Petersen, 2008). The common risk factor approach has a major benefit in that its focus is on improving health for the whole population, as well as for high risk groups.

Figure 1.10.4 shows little association between the number of DMFT among children and the number of dentists per capita. There are substantial differences in DMFT index scores among countries that have the same number of dentists per capita, indicating that many other factors affect dental health beyond the availability of dentists.

Definition and deviations

A common measure of dental health is the DMFT index. It describes the amount of dental caries in an individual through calculating the number of decayed (D), missing (M) or filled (F) permanent teeth. The sum of these three figures forms the DMFT index. In this instance, the data are for 12-year-old children. A DMFT index of less than 1.2 is judged to be very low, 1.2-2.6 is low, 2.7-4.4 is moderate, and 4.5 or more is high.

Norway provides an MFT index, which does not include decayed teeth. Sweden provides a DFT index, excluding a measure of missing teeth. The average age for New Zealand children may be slightly above 12, since Year 8 school children are surveyed. Data for Belgium and Switzerland are regional.

1.10.1 Average number of decayed, missing or filled teeth, 12-year-old children, 2006 (or latest year available)

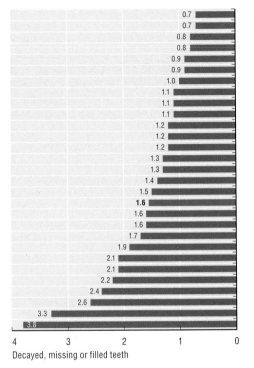

0.7	Germany (1980-2005)
0.7	United Kingdom (1983-2005)
0.8	Denmark (2006)
0.8	Luxembourg (1982-2006)
0.9	Netherlands (1980-2005)
0.9	Switzerland (1980-2005)
1.0	Sweden (1982-2005)
1.1	Australia (1980-2004)
1.1	Belgium (1983-2001)
1.1	Ireland (1980-2002)
1.2	Finland (1979-2003)
1.2	France (2006)
1.2	Italy (1980-2003)
1.3	Spain (2005)
1.3	United States (1980-2004)
1.4	Austria (1980-2007)
1.5	Portugal (1979-2006)
1.6	**OECD**
1.6	New Zealand (1980-2006)
1.6	Norway (1982-2006)
1.7	Japan (1981-2005)
1.9	Turkey (2007)
2.1	Greece (2005)
2.1	Iceland (1983-2005)
2.2	Korea (2006)
2.4	Slovak Republic (2006)
2.6	Czech Republic (2006)
3.3	Hungary (1980-2001)
3.8	Poland (1980-2000)

Decayed, missing or filled teeth

1.10.2 Decline in average number of decayed, missing or filled teeth, 12-year-old children, 1980-2006

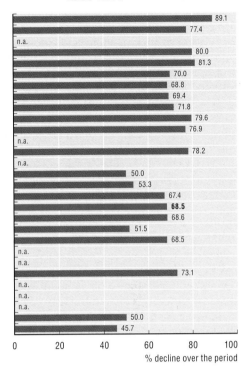
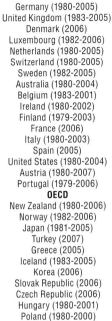

89.1	
77.4	
n.a.	
80.0	
81.3	
70.0	
68.8	
69.4	
71.8	
79.6	
76.9	
n.a.	
78.2	
n.a.	
50.0	
53.3	
67.4	
68.5	
68.6	
51.5	
68.5	
n.a.	
n.a.	
73.1	
n.a.	
n.a.	
n.a.	
50.0	
45.7	

% decline over the period

1.10.3 Average number of decayed, missing or filled teeth, 12-year-old children, selected OECD countries, 1980-2006

Germany — — — Poland — **OECD**

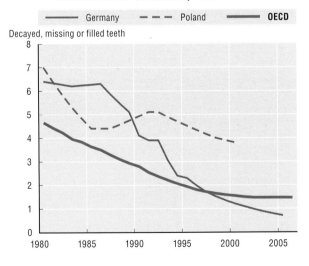

Decayed, missing or filled teeth

1.10.4 Average number of decayed, missing or filled teeth, 12-year-old children, and dentists per 1 000 population, 2006

Decayed, missing or filled teeth

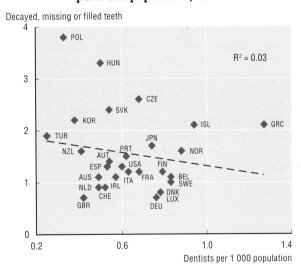

$R^2 = 0.03$

Dentists per 1 000 population

Source: OECD Health Data 2009.

StatLink ⧉ http://dx.doi.org/10.1787/717586274710

1.11. Perceived health status

Most OECD countries conduct regular health surveys which allow respondents to report on different aspects of their health. A commonly-asked question relates to self-perceived health status, of the type: "How is your health in general?". Despite the subjective nature of this question, indicators of perceived general health have been found to be a good predictor of people's future health care use and mortality (for instance, see Miilunpalo et al., 1997). For the purpose of international comparisons however, cross-country differences in perceived health status are difficult to interpret because responses may be affected by differences in the formulation of survey questions and responses, and by cultural factors.

Keeping these limitations in mind, in half of the 30 OECD countries, three-quarters or more of the adult population rate their health to be good or very good or excellent (Figure 1.11.1). New Zealand, Canada and the United States are the three countries that have the highest percentage of people assessing their health to be good or very good, with about nine out of ten people reporting to be in good health. But the response categories offered to survey respondents in these three countries are different from those used in European countries and in OECD Asian countries, which introduces an upward bias in the results (see box on "Definition and deviations" below).

In Spain and Finland, about two-thirds of the adult population rate their health to be good or very good. At the lower end of the scale, less than half of the adult population in Japan, the Slovak Republic, Portugal, Hungary and Korea rate their health to be good or very good.

Focusing on within-country differences, in the majority of countries, men are more likely than women to rate their health as good or better, and especially so in Hungary, Korea, Portugal, Spain and Turkey (Figure 1.11.2). Only in Australia, New Zealand and Finland do women rate their health as good or better more often. Unsurprisingly, people's rating of their own health tends to decline with age. In many countries, there is a particularly marked decline in a positive rating of one's own health after age 45 and a further decline after age 65. People with a lower level of education or income do not rate their health as positively as people with higher levels in all OECD countries (Mackenbach et al., 2008).

The percentage of the adult population rating their health as being good or very good has remained reasonably stable over the past 25 years in most countries where long time series are available, although some, such as Japan, have shown variation (Figure 1.11.3). The same is generally true for the population aged 65 and over. One possible interpretation of the relative stability of the indicator of perceived general health may be related to how it is measured – that is, based on a bounded variable (i.e. respondents are asked to rank their health on a five-point scale that is unchanged over time), whereas life expectancy is measured without any such limit. Another interpretation may be that people in these countries are living longer now, but possibly not healthier.

Definition and deviations

Perceived health status reflects people's overall perception of their health, and may reflect all physical and psychological dimensions. Typically, survey respondents are asked a question such as: "How is your health in general? Very good, good, fair, poor, very poor". OECD Health Data provides figures related to the proportion of people rating their health to be "good/very good" combined.

Caution is required in making cross-country comparisons of perceived health status, for at least two reasons. First, people's assessment of their health is subjective and can be affected by factors such as cultural background and national traits. Second, there are variations in the question and answer categories used to measure perceived health across surveys/countries. In particular, the response scale used in the United States, Canada, New Zealand and Australia is asymmetric (skewed on the positive side), including the following response categories: "excellent, very good, good, fair, poor". The data reported in OECD Health Data refer to respondents answering one of the three positive responses ("excellent, very good or good"). By contrast, in most other OECD countries, the response scale is symmetric, with response categories being: "very good, good, fair, poor, very poor". The data reported from these countries refer only to the first two categories ("very good, good"). Such a difference in response categories biases upward the results from those countries that are using an asymmetric scale.

1.11.1 Percentage of adults reporting to be in good health, females and males combined, 2007 (or latest year available)

1.11.2 Gender differences in the percentage of adults reporting to be in good health, 2007 (or latest year available)

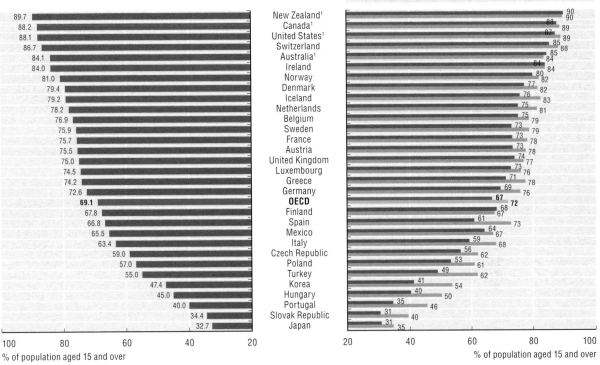

	1.11.1	1.11.2 Females	1.11.2 Males
New Zealand[1]	89.7	90	90
Canada[1]	88.2	88	89
United States[1]	88.1	87	89
Switzerland	86.7	85	88
Australia[1]	84.1	85	84
Ireland	84.0	84	84
Norway	81.0	80	82
Denmark	79.4	77	82
Iceland	79.2	76	83
Netherlands	78.2	75	81
Belgium	76.9	75	79
Sweden	75.9	73	79
France	75.7	73	78
Austria	75.5	73	78
United Kingdom	75.0	74	77
Luxembourg	74.5	73	76
Greece	74.2	71	78
Germany	72.6	69	76
OECD	**69.1**	**67**	**72**
Finland	67.8	68	67
Spain	66.8	61	73
Mexico	65.5	64	67
Italy	63.4	59	68
Czech Republic	59.0	56	62
Poland	57.0	53	61
Turkey	55.0	49	62
Korea	47.4	41	54
Hungary	45.0	40	50
Portugal	40.0	35	46
Slovak Republic	34.4	31	40
Japan	32.7	31	35

% of population aged 15 and over

% of population aged 15 and over

1. Results for these countries are not directly comparable with those for other countries, due to methodological differences in the survey questionnaire resulting in an upward bias.

1.11.3 Trends in the percentage of adults reporting to be in good health, selected OECD countries, 1980-2007

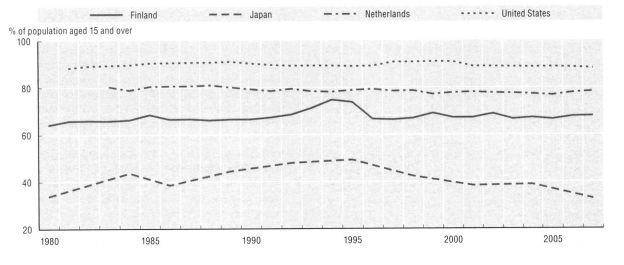

Finland — — Japan — · — Netherlands · · · · · United States

% of population aged 15 and over

Source: OECD Health Data 2009.

StatLink http://dx.doi.org/10.1787/717645721123

1.12. Diabetes prevalence and incidence

Diabetes is a chronic metabolic disease, characterised by high levels of glucose in the blood. It occurs either because the pancreas stops producing the hormone insulin (type 1 diabetes), or through a combination of the pancreas having reduced ability to produce insulin alongside the body being resistant to its action (type 2 diabetes). People with diabetes are at a greater risk of developing cardiovascular diseases such as heart attack and stroke if the disease is left undiagnosed or poorly controlled. They also have elevated risks for sight loss, foot and leg amputation due to damage to the nerves and blood vessels, and renal failure requiring dialysis or transplantation.

Diabetes was the principal cause of death of more than 300 000 persons in OECD countries in 2007, and is the fourth or fifth leading cause of death in most developed countries. However, only a minority of persons with diabetes die from diseases uniquely related to the condition – in addition, about 50% of persons with diabetes die of cardiovascular disease, and 10-20% of renal failure (IDF, 2006).

Diabetes is increasing rapidly in every part of the world, to the extent that it has now assumed epidemic proportions. Estimates suggest that more than 6% of the population aged 20-79 years in OECD countries, or 83 million people, will have diabetes in 2010. Almost half of diabetic adults are aged less than 60 years. If left unchecked, the number of people with diabetes in OECD countries will reach almost 100 million in less than 20 years (IDF, 2006).

Less than 5% of adults aged 20-79 years in Iceland, Norway and the United Kingdom will have diabetes in 2010, according to the International Diabetes Federation. This contrasts with Mexico and the United States, where more than 10% of the population of the same age have the disease (Figure 1.12.1). In most OECD countries, between 5 and 9% of the adult population have diabetes.

Type 1 diabetes accounts for only 10-15% of all diabetes cases. It is the predominant form of the disease in younger age groups in most developed countries. Based on disease registers and recent studies, the annual number of new cases of type 1 diabetes in children aged under 15 years is high at 25 or more per 100 000 population in Nordic countries (Finland, Sweden and Norway) (Figure 1.12.2). Korea, Mexico, Japan and Turkey have less than five new cases per 100 000 population. Alarmingly, there is evidence that type 1 diabetes is developing at an earlier age among children (IDF, 2006).

The economic impact of diabetes is substantial. Health expenditure to treat and prevent diabetes and its complications was estimated at USD 212 billion in OECD countries in 2007 (IDF, 2006). In the United States alone, some USD 116 billion was spent on care to treat diabetes, along with its complications and excess general medical costs in 2007 (ADA, 2008). In Australia, direct health care expenditure on diabetes in 2004-05 accounted for nearly 2% of the recurrent health expenditure (AIHW, 2008d). Around one-quarter of medical expenditure is spent on controlling elevated blood glucose, another quarter on treating long-term complication of diabetes, and the remainder on additional general medical care (IDF, 2006). Increasing costs reinforce the need to provide quality care for the management of diabetes and its complications (see Indicator 5.2 "Avoidable admissions: diabetes complications").

Type 2 diabetes is largely preventable. A number of risk factors, such as overweight and obesity and physical inactivity are modifiable, and can also help reduce the complications that are associated with diabetes. But in most countries, the prevalence of overweight and obesity also continues to increase (see Indicator 2.7 "Overweight and obesity among adults").

Definition and deviations

The sources and methods used by the International Diabetes Federation for publishing national prevalence estimates of diabetes are outlined in their *Diabetes Atlas, 4th edition* (IDF, 2009). Country data were derived from studies published between 1980 and February 2009, and were only included if they met several criteria for reliability.

Studies from several OECD countries – Canada, France, Italy, Netherlands, Norway and the United Kingdom – only provided self-reported data on diabetes. To account for undiagnosed diabetes, the prevalence of diabetes for Canada and the United Kingdom was multiplied by a factor of 1.5, in accordance with findings from the United States (for Canada) and local recommendations (for the United Kingdom), and doubled for other countries, based on data from a number of countries.

Prevalence rates were adjusted to the World Standard Population to facilitate cross-national comparisons.

1.12.1 Prevalence estimates of diabetes, adults aged 20-79 years, 2010

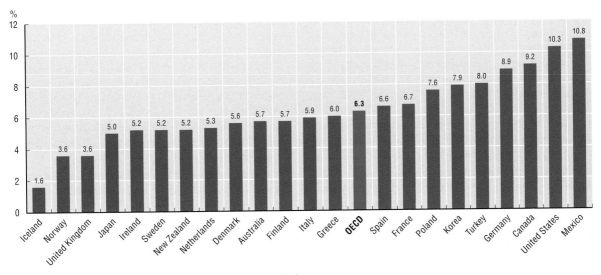

Note: The data are age-standardised to the World Standard Population.

1.12.2 Incidence estimates of Type 1 diabetes, children aged 0-14 years, 2010

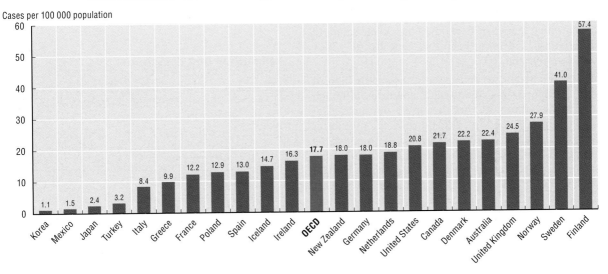

Source: IDF (2009).

StatLink ⌐⌐⌐ http://dx.doi.org/10.1787/717657703771

The first cases of Acquired Immunodeficiency Syndrome (AIDS) were diagnosed almost 30 years ago. The onset of AIDS is normally caused as a result of HIV (human immunodeficiency virus) infection and can manifest itself as any number of different diseases, such as pneumonia and tuberculosis, as the immune system is no longer able to defend the body. There is a time lag between HIV infection, AIDS diagnosis and death due to HIV infection, which can be any number of years depending on the treatment administered. Despite worldwide research, there is no cure currently available.

In 2006, the number of reported new cases of AIDS stood at approximately 45 000 across the OECD area as a whole, representing an unweighted average incidence rate of 16.2 per million population (Figure 1.13.1). Since the first reporting of AIDS cases in the early 1980s, the number of cases rose rapidly to reach an average of more than 45 new cases per million population across OECD countries at its peak in the first half of the 1990s, almost three times current incidence rates (Figure 1.13.2). Public awareness campaigns contributed to steady declines in reported cases through the second half of the 1990s. In addition, the development and greater availability of antiretroviral drugs, which reduce or slow down the development of the disease, led to a sharp decrease in incidence between 1996 and 1997.

The United States has consistently shown the highest AIDS incidence rates among OECD countries, although it is important to note that the case reporting definitions were expanded in 1993 and subsequently differ from the definition used across Europe and other OECD countries. The change in definition also explains the large increase in cases in the United States in 1993 (Figure 1.13.2). In Europe, Spain reported the highest incidence rates in the first decade following the outbreak, although there has been a sharp decline since 1994, leaving Portugal currently with the highest rate among European countries. Central European countries such as the Czech and Slovak Republics and Hungary, along with Turkey, Korea and Japan report the lowest incidence rates of AIDS among OECD countries.

In the United States, over one million people are currently living with HIV/AIDS, including over 450 000 with AIDS (CDC, 2008). Almost three-quarters of new cases of AIDS diagnosed in 2006 were among men, and racial and ethnic minorities continue to be disproportionately affected by the epidemic. In Canada, Aboriginal people are over-represented. In most OECD countries, the main risk factor for HIV infection remains unprotected sex between men. Approximately 75% of heterosexually acquired HIV infection in western and central Europe is among migrants.

In recent years, the overall decline in AIDS cases has slowed down. This reversal has been accompanied by evidence of increasing transmission of HIV in several European countries (ECDC and WHO, 2008), attributed to complacency regarding the effectiveness of treatment and a waning of public awareness regarding drug use and sexual practice. Further inroads in AIDS incidence rates will require more intensive HIV prevention programmes that are focused and adapted to reach those most at risk of HIV infection (UNAIDS, 2008).

Definition and deviations

The incidence rate of AIDS is the number of new cases per million population at year of diagnosis. Note that data for recent years are provisional due to reporting delays, which sometimes can be for several years depending on the country.

The United States expanded their AIDS surveillance case definition in 1993 to include T-lymphocyte count criteria. This broadening of the definition led to a large increase in the number of new cases in the United States in 1993 and explains some of the current variations in AIDS incidence between the United States and other OECD countries.

1.13.1 AIDS incidence rates, 2006

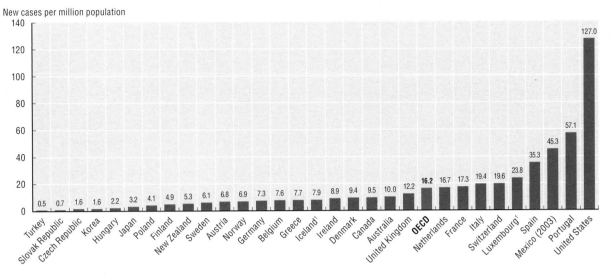

1. Three-year average (2004-06).

1.13.2 Trends in AIDS incidence rates, selected OECD countries, 1981-2006

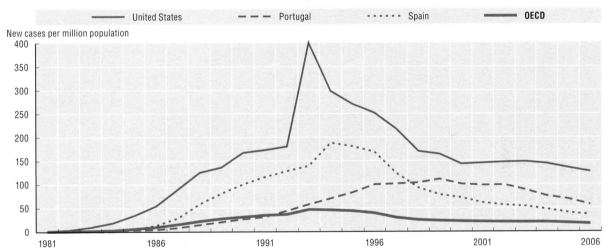

Note: The United States expanded their AIDS surveillance case definition in 1993.

Source: OECD Health Data 2009. Data for European countries are extracted from the ECDC and WHO Regional Office for Europe (2008), "HIV/AIDS surveillance in Europe, 2007".

StatLink ᐅᐧᐨ *http://dx.doi.org/10.1787/717661732382*

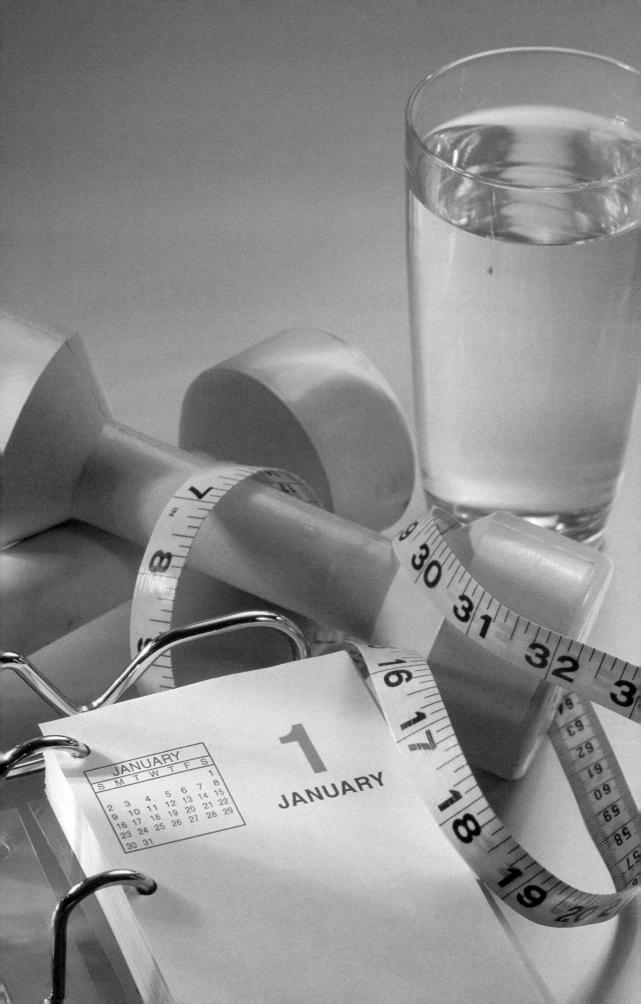

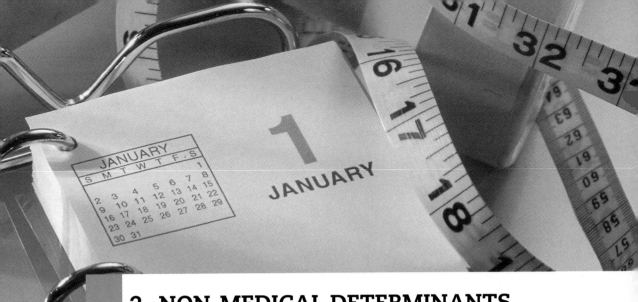

2. NON-MEDICAL DETERMINANTS OF HEALTH

Regular smoking or excessive drinking in adolescence has immediate and long-term health consequences. Children who establish smoking habits in early adolescence increase their risk of cardiovascular diseases, respiratory illnesses and cancer. They are also more likely to experiment with alcohol and other drugs. Alcohol misuse is itself associated with a range of social, physical and mental health problems, including depressive and anxiety disorders, obesity and accidental injury (Currie *et al.*, 2008).

Results from the Health Behaviour in School-aged Children (HBSC) surveys, a series of collaborative cross-national studies conducted in most OECD countries, allow for monitoring of smoking and drinking behaviours among adolescents. Generally, today girls smoke more than boys, but more boys get drunk. Between 13 and 15 years of age, the prevalence of smoking and drunkenness doubles in many OECD countries.

Children in Austria, Finland, Hungary, the Czech Republic and Italy smoke more often, with weekly rates of 20% or more for both boys and girls (Figure 2.1.1). In contrast, 10% or less of 15-year-olds in the United States, Canada and Sweden smoke weekly. Most countries report higher rates of smoking for girls, although only Spain and Austria have differences in excess of 5%. Greece, Finland, Hungary, Iceland, Poland and the Slovak Republic are the only countries where smoking is more prevalent among boys.

Drunkenness at least twice in their lifetime is reported by 40% or more of 15-year-olds in Denmark, the United Kingdom and Finland (Figure 2.1.2). Across all surveyed countries, 29% of girls and 33% of boys have been drunk on two or more occasions, with much lower rates in the United States, and Mediterranean countries such as Greece, Italy and Portugal. Boys are more likely to report repeated drunkenness. Switzerland, Belgium, Hungary and the Slovak Republic have the biggest differences, with rates of alcohol abuse being 5-10% higher than those of girls. In Poland, differences are even greater, with repeated drunkenness among boys being over 10% higher than girls. Norway, Spain, Canada and the United Kingdom are the only countries where more girls report repeated drunkenness, and in each case rates are less than 5% higher.

The differences in recent smoking and drinking rates between 15-year-old boys and girls are shown in Figure 2.1.3. Countries above the 45 degree line have

higher rates for girls, and countries below the line higher rates for boys. Countries with higher rates of smoking among boys also report higher rates for girls, with the same finding for drinking rates.

Rates of drunkenness are also available for 13-year-olds (Currie *et al.*, 2008). At this age, over one in ten children in the United Kingdom, Finland, Canada and the Slovak Republic have experienced drunkenness more than twice. In Poland and Hungary, high rates of repeated drunkenness at 13 are also seen for boys. The largest relative increase in reported drunkenness between the ages of 13 and 15 are seen in Norway, Iceland and Sweden, but the rate in each of these countries remains below average at age 15.

Risk-taking behaviours among adolescents are falling, with both alcohol and cigarette consumption among 15-year-olds showing some decline from the levels of the late 1990s (Figure 2.1.4). With the exception of Greece, all surveyed OECD countries report falling rates of smoking for both boys and girls. Levels of smoking for both sexes are at their lowest for a decade with, on average, fewer than one in five children of either sex smoking regularly. Some country convergence in risk behaviours is also evident: among girls for smoking, and drunkenness for both boys and girls.

Definition and deviations

Estimates for smoking refer to the proportion of 15-year-old children who self-report smoking at least once a week. Estimates for drunkenness record the proportions of 13- and 15-year-old children saying they have been drunk more than twice in their lives.

Data for 24 OECD countries are from Health Behaviour in School-aged Children (HBSC) surveys undertaken between 1992-93 and 2005-06. Data are drawn from school-based samples. France, Germany and the United Kingdom report results for certain regions only. The survey has not been carried out in Australia, Japan, Korea, Mexico and New Zealand. Turkey is included in the 2005-06 HBSC survey, but did not question children on drinking and smoking.

2.1.1 Smoking among 15-year-olds, 2005-06

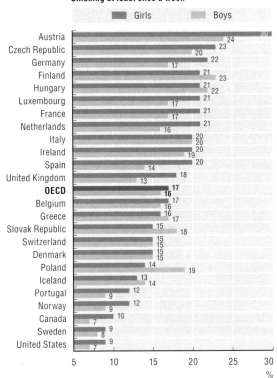

Source: Currie et al. (2008).

2.1.2 Drunkenness among 15-year-olds, 2005-06

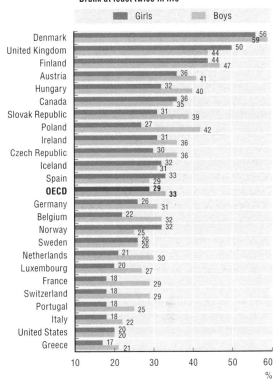

2.1.3 Risk behaviours of 15-year-olds, by sex, 2005-06

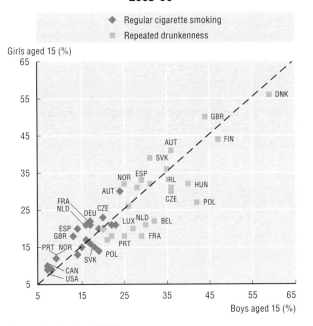

Source: Currie et al. (2008).

2.1.4 Trends in repeated drunkenness and regular smoking among 15-year-olds, OECD average

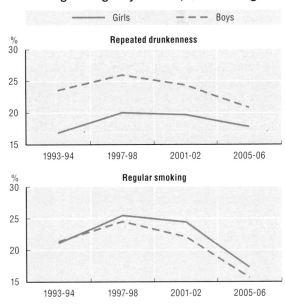

Source: Currie et al. (2000, 2004, 2008); WHO (1996).

StatLink ⟨⟨⟨ http://dx.doi.org/10.1787/717673302465

Nutrition is important for children's development and long-term health. Eating fruit during adolescence, for example, in place of high-fat, sugar and salt products, can protect against health problems such as obesity, diabetes, and heart problems. Moreover, eating fruit when young can be habit forming, promoting healthy eating behaviours for later life.

A number of factors influence the amount of fruit consumed by adolescents, including family income, the cost of alternatives, preparation time, whether parents eat fruit, and the availability of fresh fruit which can be linked to the country or local climate (Rasmussen *et al.*, 2006). Low family affluence is associated with lower fruit consumption in most OECD countries. Fruit (and vegetable) consumption have a high priority as indicators of healthy eating in most OECD countries.

In 2005-06, only around one-third of boys and two-fifths of girls aged 11-15 years ate at least one piece of fruit daily, according to the latest Health Behaviour in School-aged Children (HBSC) survey (Currie *et al.*, 2008). Overall, boys in Italy, and girls in the United Kingdom had the highest rates of daily fruit consumption. Fruit consumption is relatively low among some Nordic countries, including Finland, Iceland and Sweden. Finnish children reported the lowest levels of daily fruit consumption, with rates lower than one in four girls and one in five boys. Girls at all ages in most countries were more likely to eat fruit daily. At age 11, girls in Norway, Portugal and Switzerland, as well as boys in Portugal, the United States and Italy were more likely to eat fruit daily. By age 15, girls in Italy, Denmark and the United Kingdom, and boys in Italy, Portugal and Belgium ate most (Figure 2.2.1).

In almost all OECD countries, daily fruit consumption falls between ages 11 and 15 (Figure 2.2.2). Among girls, the OECD average fell from 46% at age 11, to 40% at age 13 and 36% at age 15. For boys, the fall was from 38% to 33% and then 26%. In Austria and Iceland, rates fell by up to half between ages 11 and 15, and severe falls were also seen in Hungary (girls). Italy (girls), as well as Belgium (boys) are the most successful coun-

tries in maintaining healthy eating habits as children get older.

The gap between the fruit consumption of boys and girls is largest at age 15, for most countries. At age 11, France, Italy and Spain are most equal in terms of fruit eating by sex. Norway, Germany and Poland have the biggest gaps at this age. As children reach age 15, gaps in Denmark, the Czech Republic and Turkey grow to a level where fewer than six boys for every ten girls eat fruit regularly.

Average reported rates of daily fruit consumption across OECD countries showed some increase between 2001-02 and 2005-06. This was most evident among girls aged 11 (Figure 2.2.3).

Effective strategies are required in order to ensure that children are eating enough fruit to conform with recommended dietary guidelines. Children generally hold a positive attitude toward fruit intake, and report good availability of fruit at home, but lower availability at school and during leisure time. Increased accessibility to fruit, combined with educational and motivational activities, can help in increasing fruit consumption (Sandvik *et al.*, 2005).

Definition and deviations

Nutrition is measured in terms of the proportions of children who report eating fruit at least every day or more than once a day. In addition to fruit, healthy nutrition also involves other types of foods.

Data for 25 OECD countries are from the Health Behaviour in School-aged Children (HBSC) surveys undertaken in 2001-02 and 2005-06. Data are drawn from school-based samples. France, Germany and the United Kingdom report results for certain regions only. The survey has not been carried out in Australia, Japan, Korea, Mexico and New Zealand.

2.2.1 Daily fruit eating among 11 and 15-year-olds, 2005-06

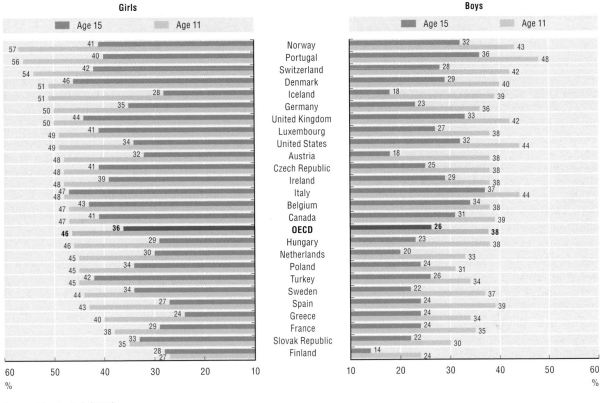

Source: Currie et al. (2008).

2.2.2 Regular fruit consumption at ages 11 and 15 by sex, 2005-06

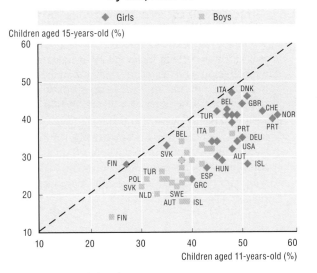

Source: Currie et al. (2008).

2.2.3 Average proportion of children reporting daily fruit consumption, by sex, 2001-02 and 2005-06

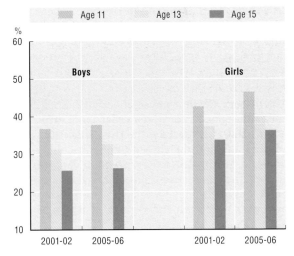

Source: Currie et al. (2004, 2008).

StatLink ⬛⬛ http://dx.doi.org/10.1787/717755520653

Undertaking physical activity in adolescence is beneficial for health, and can set standards for adult physical activity levels, thereby indirectly influencing health outcomes in later life. Research supports the role that physical activity in adolescence has in the prevention and treatment of a range of youth health issues including asthma, mental health, bone health and obesity. More direct links to adult health are found between physical activity in adolescence and its effect on overweight and obesity and related diseases, breast cancer rates and bone health in later life. The health effects of adolescent physical activity are largely dependent on the activity type, *e.g.* water physical activities in adolescence are effective in the treatment of asthma, and exercise is recommended in the treatment of cystic fibrosis (Hallal *et al.*, 2006; Currie *et al.*, 2008).

Some of the factors influencing the levels of physical activity undertaken by adolescents include the availability of space and equipment, the child's present health conditions, their school curricula and other competing pastimes.

One in five children in OECD countries undertake moderate-to-vigorous exercise regularly, according to results from the 2005-06 HBSC survey (Figure 2.3.1). Children in Switzerland and France are least likely to exercise regularly, whereas the Slovak Republic and Ireland stand out as strong performers with over 40 and 30% respectively of children aged 11 to 15 exercising for a total of at least 60 minutes per day over the past week. The country rankings reported vary according to the child's age. France appears at the lower end, especially for girls, at all ages. There is very little change in the rates of exercise among boys in the United States at ages 11, 13 and 15, with one in three children meeting the recommended guidelines throughout all ages. Boys consistently undertake more physical activity than girls, across all countries and all age groups.

It is of concern that physical activity tends to fall between ages 11 to 15 for most OECD countries (Figure 2.3.2), with boys in the Czech Republic, Luxembourg and the United States the only exceptions. In Portugal, Norway, Sweden, Austria, and Finland, the rates of exercising among boys more than halve between ages 11 and 15. The rates of girls exercising to recommended levels also falls between

the ages of 11 and 15 years. In the Czech Republic, Luxembourg, Belgium, and Switzerland, rates for 15-year-old girls fall to as little as one-fifth of those reported at age 11. Similarly, in Iceland, Ireland and Finland, rates of physical activity among girls fall by over 60%.

To compare levels of exercise between 2001-02 and 2005-06, results are reported in relation to the OECD average (Figure 2.3.3). In 2001-02, rates refer to children reporting an hour of moderate to vigorous exercise five days a week, but in 2005-06 figures refer to exercise of this type seven days a week. Boys' rates were above the OECD average in the Netherlands, Austria, the United Kingdom, Poland and Greece in 2001-02, but fell below the average in 2005-06. Finland, Hungary, and Denmark are countries where rates of physical activity were below the OECD average in 2001-02, but were among the higher performers in 2005-06. For boys, only Ireland, the United States and Canada have been consistently high performers on measures of physical activity in both waves. For girls, Spain and Belgium have moved from below average performances in 2001-02 to above average in 2005-06. In Sweden, Poland, the United Kingdom, and Austria, rates of physical activity among girls have fallen below the OECD average since 2001-02.

Definition and deviations

Data for physical activity considers the regularity of moderate-to-vigorous physical activity as reported by 11-, 13- and 15-year-olds for the years 2001-02 and 2005-06. Moderate-to-vigorous physical activity refers to exercise undertaken for at least an hour which increases both heart rate and respiration (and leaves the child out of breath sometimes) on five or more days per week in 2001-02, and seven days a week in 2005-06.

Indicators are taken from the Health Behaviour in School-aged Children Survey (HBSC). Data are drawn from school-based samples, but some countries report regional results only. The survey was not carried out in Australia, Japan, Korea, Mexico and New Zealand.

2.3.1 Children aged 11-15 years doing moderate-to-vigorous physical activity daily in the past week, 2005-06

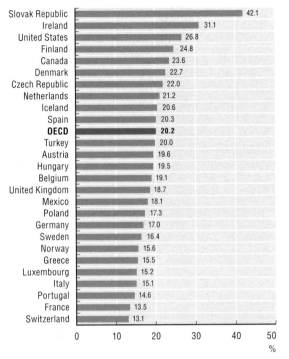

	%
Slovak Republic	42.1
Ireland	31.1
United States	26.8
Finland	24.8
Canada	23.6
Denmark	22.7
Czech Republic	22.0
Netherlands	21.2
Iceland	20.6
Spain	20.3
OECD	**20.2**
Turkey	20.0
Austria	19.6
Hungary	19.5
Belgium	19.1
United Kingdom	18.7
Mexico	18.1
Poland	17.3
Germany	17.0
Sweden	16.4
Norway	15.6
Greece	15.5
Luxembourg	15.2
Italy	15.1
Portugal	14.6
France	13.5
Switzerland	13.1

2.3.2 Comparing physical activity of 11- and 15-year-old children by sex, 2005-06

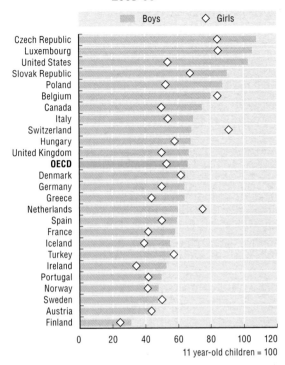

11 year-old children = 100

2.3.3 Standardised rates of physical activity (OECD average = 1) by sex, 2001-02 and 2005-06

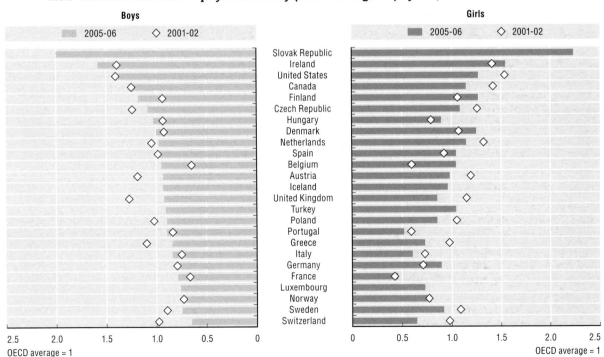

Source: Currie et al. (2004, 2008).

StatLink ᔡᔥᒪ http://dx.doi.org/10.1787/717758031100

Children who are overweight or obese are at greater risk of poor health in adolescence and in adulthood. Being overweight in childhood increases the risk of developing cardiovascular disease or diabetes, as well as related social and mental health problems. Excess weight problems in childhood are associated with an increased risk of being an obese adult, where certain forms of cancer, osteoarthritis, a reduced quality of life and premature death can be added to the list of health concerns (Currie *et al.*, 2008; WHO Europe, 2007).

Evidence suggests that even if excess childhood weight is lost, adults who were obese children retain an increased risk of cardiovascular problems. And although dieting can combat obesity, children who diet are at a greater risk of putting on weight following periods of dieting. Eating disorders, symptoms of stress and postponed physical development can also be products of dieting.

Across most OECD countries, one in seven children are overweight or obese (Figure 2.4.1). Aggregate figures for 2005-06 show that nearly one in three children in the United States, and one in five in Canada, are overweight or obese – the highest rates among surveyed countries in the OECD. Southern European countries such as Portugal, Greece, Italy and Spain also have higher rates of children with excess weight problems. Fewer than one in ten children in the Netherlands, Switzerland, the Slovak Republic and Denmark are overweight or obese.

There is no clear association between weight problems and weight reduction behaviours at the national level. In most countries, the number of children trying to lose weight is greater than the number with excess weight problems. Generally, countries where few children report excess weight problems also report weight reduction behaviours close to the OECD average. The six countries with the highest rates of overweight and obese children have similar levels of weight reduction behaviour, each around the OECD average of 14%, even though the proportion of children with excess weight problems varies widely.

There are important differences among children with excess weight problems, according to their age. In some countries older children have more excess weight than younger children, for others countries the opposite is true (Figure 2.4.2). Countries in the top right hand corner of the figure report cohort changes above the OECD average for both boys and girls. A number of countries, including the Netherlands, Norway, Sweden, Iceland and Switzerland report increases in overweight and obesity rates for both boys and girls as children get older. Eight countries

have below average differences for both boys and girls. The Czech Republic stands out as the only country where rates of excess weight for both boys and girls are lower for the 15-year-old cohorts compared to the 11-year-old cohorts

Rates of overweight and obese boys and girls are increasing across the OECD (Figure 2.4.3). Between 2001-02 and 2005-06, every surveyed country reported an increase in overweight or obesity for boys aged 15. The largest increases during the four year period were found in the United States, Portugal and Austria. A similar pattern of increases is seen for girls, with rates in the United States, Portugal and Germany almost doubling. Only Ireland and the United Kingdom report reductions in the proportion of overweight or obese girls at age 15 between 2001-02 and 2005-06. However, because non-response rates to questions of self-reported height and weight were high in both these countries, cautious interpretation is required.

Definition and deviations

Estimates of overweight and obesity are based on Body Mass Index (BMI) calculations using child self-reported height and weight. Overweight and obese children are those whose BMI is above a set of age- and sex-specific cut-off points (Cole *et al.*, 2000). Data on weight reduction record children who report being on a diet or doing something else to lose weight.

Self-reported height and weight is subject to under-reporting and error, and requires cautious interpretation. In 2005-06, Canada, England and Norway have missing data for over 30% of respondents for 11-year-olds. The same is true for England, Ireland and Belgium for 13-years-olds, and in England and Ireland for 15-year-olds. In 2001-02, BMI data are missing for over 30% of respondents in Ireland.

Indicators are taken from the Health Behaviour in School-aged Children Surveys in 2001-02 and 2005-06. Aggregate country estimates are crude rates of overweight and obese 11-, 13- and 15-year-olds in each country. Some countries report regional data only. Data are drawn from school-based samples. The survey was not carried out in Australia, Japan, Korea, Mexico and New Zealand.

2.4.1 Children aged 11-15 years who are overweight or obese, and children who are involved in weight-reduction behaviour, 2005-06

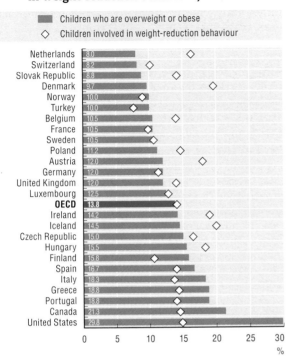

2.4.2 Percentage difference in obesity rates between 11 and 15 years by sex, 2005-06

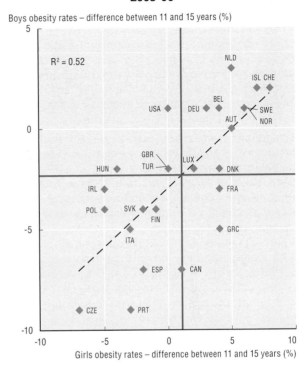

Note: The red lines represent the OECD average.

2.4.3 Change in obesity rates between 2001-02 and 2005-06, for 15-year-old boys and girls

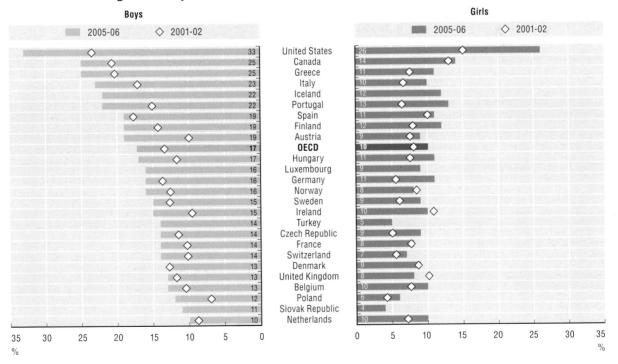

Source: Currie et al. (2004, 2008).

StatLink ᔆ᠊ᘓᔆ᠊ http://dx.doi.org/10.1787/717762448712

2.5. Tobacco consumption among adults

Tobacco is the second major cause of death in the world, after cardiovascular disease, and is directly responsible for about one in ten adult deaths worldwide, equating to about 6 million deaths each year (Shafey *et al.*, 2009). It is a major risk factor for at least two of the leading causes of premature mortality – circulatory diseases and a range of cancers. In addition, it is an important contributory factor for respiratory diseases, while smoking among pregnant women can lead to low birth weight and illnesses among infants. It remains the largest avoidable risk to health in OECD countries.

The proportion of daily smokers among the adult population varies greatly across countries, even between neighboring countries (Figure 2.5.1). In 2007, rates were lowest in Sweden, the United States, Australia, New Zealand, Canada, Iceland and Portugal, all at less than 20% of the adult population smoking daily. On average, smoking rates have decreased by about 5 percentage points in OECD countries since 1995, with a higher decline in men than in women. Large declines occurred in Turkey (47% to 33%), Luxembourg (33% to 21%), Norway (33% to 22%), Japan (37% to 26%) and Denmark (36% to 25%). Greece maintains the highest level of smoking, along with Turkey and Hungary, with 30% or more of the adult population smoking daily. Greece and Mexico are the only OECD countries where smoking appears to be increasing in both men and women.

In the post-war period, most OECD countries tended to follow a general pattern marked by very high smoking rates among men (50% or more) through to the 1960s and 1970s, while the 1980s and the 1990s were characterised by a marked downturn in tobacco consumption. Much of this decline can be attributed to policies aimed at reducing tobacco consumption through public awareness campaigns, advertising bans and increased taxation, in response to rising rates of tobacco-related diseases (World Bank, 1999). In addition to government policies, actions by anti-smoking interest groups were very effective in reducing smoking rates by changing beliefs about the health effects of smoking, particularly in North America (Cutler and Glaeser, 2006).

Although large disparities remain, smoking rates across most OECD countries have shown a marked decline over recent decades (Figure 2.5.3). Smoking prevalence among men continues to be higher than among women in all OECD countries except Sweden

and Norway. Female smoking rates continue to decline in most OECD countries, and in a number of cases (Turkey, New Zealand, Iceland, Canada, United States, United Kingdom and Ireland) at an even faster pace than male rates. Only in five countries do female smoking rates appear to have been increasing over the last 12 years (Austria, Germany, Greece, Mexico and Portugal), but in these countries women are still less likely to smoke than men. In 2007, the gender gap in smoking rates was particularly large in Korea, Japan and Turkey and, to a lesser extent, in Mexico, Portugal, Greece and Poland (Figure 2.5.2).

Several studies provide strong evidence of socio-economic differences in smoking and mortality (Mackenbach *et al.*, 2008). People in lower social groups have a greater prevalence and intensity of smoking, a higher all-cause mortality rate and lower rates of cancer survival (Woods *et al.*, 2006). The influence of smoking as a determinant of overall health inequalities is such that, in a non-smoking population, mortality differences between social groups would be halved (Jha *et al.*, 2006).

Figure 2.5.4 shows the correlation between tobacco consumption (as measured by grams per capita) and incidence of lung cancer across OECD countries, with a time lag of two decades. Higher tobacco consumption at the national level is also generally associated with higher mortality rates from lung cancer one or two decades later across OECD countries.

Definition and deviations

The proportion of daily smokers is defined as the percentage of the population aged 15 years and over reporting smoking every day.

International comparability is limited due to the lack of standardisation in the measurement of smoking habits in health interview surveys across OECD countries. Variations remain in the wording of questions, response categories and survey methodologies, *e.g.* in a number of countries, respondents are asked if they smoke regularly, rather than daily.

2.5.1 Percentage of adult population smoking daily, 2007 (or latest year available)

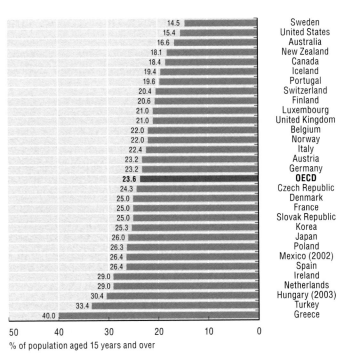

% of population aged 15 years and over

2.5.2 Percentage of females and males smoking daily, 2007 (or latest year available)

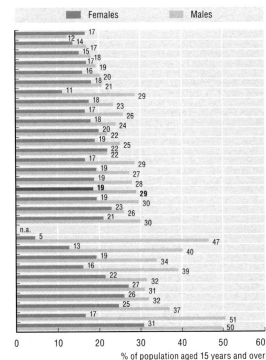

% of population aged 15 years and over

2.5.3 Change in smoking rates by gender, 1995-2007 (or nearest year)

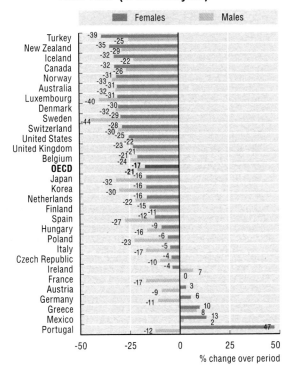

% change over period

2.5.4 Tobacco consumption, 1980 and incidence of lung cancer, 2002

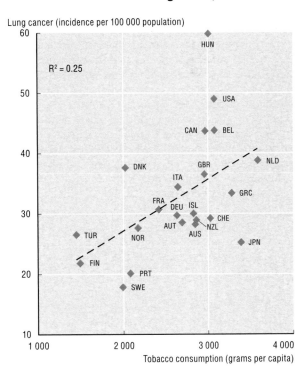

Source: OECD Health Data 2009.

StatLink http://dx.doi.org/10.1787/717778312610

2.6. Alcohol consumption among adults

The global health burden related to excessive alcohol consumption, both in terms of morbidity and mortality, is considerable in most parts of the world (Rehm *et al.*, 2009; WHO, 2004b). It is associated with numerous harmful health and social consequences, including drunkenness and alcohol dependence. High alcohol intake increases the risk for heart, stroke and vascular diseases, as well as liver cirrhosis and certain cancers. Foetal exposure to alcohol increases the risk of birth defects and intellectual impairments. Alcohol also contributes to death and disability through accidents and injuries, assault, violence, homicide and suicide, and is estimated to cause more than 2 million deaths annually. It is, however, one of the major avoidable risk factors for disease.

Alcohol consumption, as measured by annual sales, stands on average across OECD countries at 9.7 litres per adult, using the most recent data available. Leaving aside Luxembourg – given the high volume of purchases by non-residents in that country – Ireland, Hungary and France reported the highest consumption of alcohol, with 13.0 litres or more per adult per year in 2006-07. At the other end of the scale, Turkey, Mexico and some of the Nordic countries (Norway and Sweden) have relatively low levels of alcohol consumption, ranging from one to seven litres per adult (Figure 2.6.1).

Although average alcohol consumption has gradually fallen in many OECD countries over the past two decades, it has risen in some others (Figure 2.6.2). There has been a degree of convergence in drinking habits across the OECD, with wine consumption increasing in many traditional beer-drinking countries and *vice versa*. The traditional wine-producing countries of Italy, France and Spain, as well as the Slovak Republic and Greece, have seen their alcohol consumption per capita drop substantially since 1980 (Figures 2.6.2 and 2.6.3). On the other hand, alcohol consumption per capita in Iceland, Ireland and Mexico rose by as much as 40% or more since 1980 although, in the case of Iceland and Mexico, it started from a very low level and therefore remains relatively low.

Variations in alcohol consumption across countries and over time reflect not only changing drinking habits but also the policy responses to control alcohol use. Curbs on advertising, sales restrictions and taxation have all proven to be effective measures to reduce alcohol consumption (Bennett, 2003). Strict controls on sales and high taxation are mirrored by overall lower consumption in most Nordic countries, while falls in consumption in France, Italy and Spain may be associated with the voluntary and statutory regulation of advertising, partly following a 1989 European directive.

Although adult alcohol consumption per capita gives useful evidence of long-term trends, it does not identify sub-populations at risk from harmful drinking patterns. The consumption of large quantities of alcohol at a single session, termed "binge drinking", is a particularly dangerous pattern of consumption (Institute of Alcohol Studies, 2007), which is on the rise in some countries and social groups, especially among young males (see Indicator 2.1 "Smoking and alcohol consumption at age 15").

Figure 2.6.4 shows the relationship between alcohol consumption in 1990 and deaths from liver cirrhosis in 2006. In general, countries with high levels of alcohol consumption tend to experience higher death rates from liver cirrhosis 10 to 15 years later compared with countries with lower levels of consumption. In most OECD countries, death rates from liver cirrhosis have fallen over the past two decades, following quite closely the overall reduction in alcohol consumption.

Definition and deviations

Alcohol consumption is defined as annual sales of pure alcohol in litres per person aged 15 years and over. The methodology to convert alcohol drinks to pure alcohol may differ across countries.

Italy reports consumption for the population 14 years and over, Sweden for 16 years and over, and Japan 20 years and over. In some countries (*e.g.* Luxembourg), national sales do not accurately reflect actual consumption by residents, since purchases by non-residents may create a significant gap between national sales and consumption.

2.6.1 Alcohol consumption, population aged 15 years and over, 2007 (or latest year available)

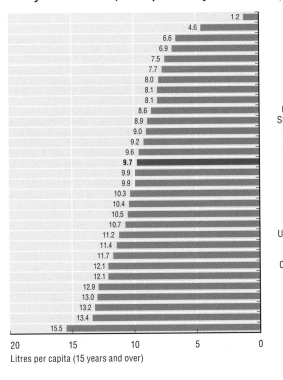

2.6.2 Change in alcohol consumption per capita, population aged 15 years and over, 1980-2007

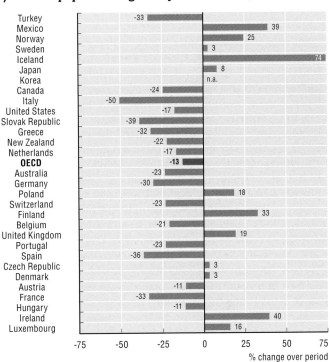

2.6.3 Trends in alcohol consumption, selected OECD countries, 1980-2007

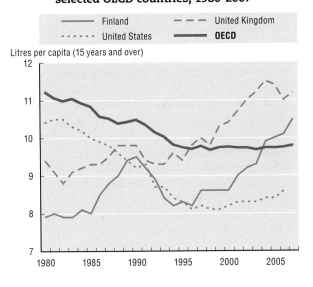

2.6.4 Alcohol consumption, 1990 and liver cirrhosis deaths, 2006

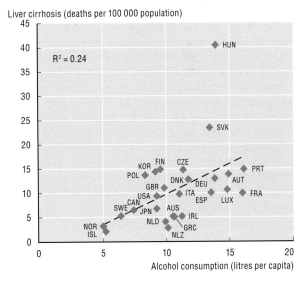

Source: OECD Health Data 2009.

StatLink ⫿⫿⧠ *http://dx.doi.org/10.1787/717840061754*

The growth in overweight and obesity rates among adults is a major public health concern. Obesity is a known risk factor for numerous health problems, including hypertension, high cholesterol, diabetes, cardiovascular diseases, respiratory problems (asthma), musculoskeletal diseases (arthritis) and some forms of cancer.

Half or more of the adult population is now defined as being either overweight or obese in no less than 13 OECD countries: Mexico, United States, United Kingdom, Australia, Greece, New Zealand, Luxembourg, Hungary, Czech Republic, Portugal, Ireland, Spain and Iceland. In contrast, overweight and obesity rates are much lower in Japan and Korea and in some European countries (France and Switzerland), although rates are also increasing in these countries. The prevalence of obesity (which presents greater health risks than overweight) varies tenfold among OECD countries, from a low of 3% in Japan and Korea, to over 30% in the United States and Mexico (Figures 2.7.1 and 2.7.2).

The rate of obesity has more than doubled over the past 20 years in the United States, while it has almost tripled in Australia and more than tripled in the United Kingdom (Figure 2.7.3). Some 20-24% of adults in the United Kingdom, Australia, Iceland and Luxembourg are obese, about the same rate as in the United States in the early 1990s. Obesity rates in many western European countries have increased substantially over the past decade.

In many countries, the rise in obesity has affected all population groups, regardless of sex, age, race, income or education level. Evidence from nine OECD countries (Australia, Austria, Canada, England, France, Italy, Korea, Spain and the United States) indicates that obesity tends to be more common among individuals in disadvantaged socio-economic groups, particularly among women (Sassi et al., 2009b). Also, an examination of four OECD countries (Australia, Canada, England and Korea) shows a broadly linear relationship between the number of years spent in full-time education and obesity, with the most educated individuals displaying lower rates. Again, the gradient in obesity is stronger in women than in men (Sassi et al., 2009a).

Because obesity is associated with higher risks of chronic illnesses, it is linked to significant additional health care costs. It has been estimated that health care costs which might be attributed to obesity accounted for about 5-7% of total health spending in the United States in the late 1990s, and to 3.5% of health spending in other countries such as Canada, Australia and New Zealand (Thompson and Wolf, 2001). There is a time lag between the onset of obesity and related health problems, suggesting that the rise in obesity over the past two decades will mean higher health care costs in the future. A recent study estimated that total costs linked to overweight and obesity in England in 2015 could increase by as much as 70% relative to 2007 and could be 2.4 times higher in 2025 (Foresight, 2007).

A number of behavioural and environmental factors have contributed to the rise in overweight and obesity rates in industrialised countries, including falling real prices of food and more time spent being physically inactive. Overweight and obesity has risen rapidly in children in recent decades, reaching double-figure rates in most OECD countries (see also Indicator 2.4 "Overweight and obesity among children").

Definition and deviations

Overweight and obesity are defined as excessive weight presenting health risks because of the high proportion of body fat. The most frequently used measure is based on the Body Mass Index (BMI), which is a single number that evaluates an individual's weight in relation to height (weight/height^2, with weight in kilograms and height in metres). Based on the WHO classification (WHO, 2000), adults with a BMI between 25 and 30 are defined as overweight, and those with a BMI over 30 as obese. This classification may not be suitable for all ethnic groups, who may have equivalent levels of risk at lower or higher BMI. The thresholds for adults are not suitable to measure overweight and obesity among children.

For most countries, overweight and obesity rates are self-reported through estimates of height and weight from population-based health interview surveys. The exceptions are Australia, Czech Republic (2005), Japan, Luxembourg, New Zealand, the Slovak Republic (2007), the United Kingdom and the United States, where estimates are derived from health examinations. These differences limit data comparability. Estimates from health examinations are generally higher and more reliable than from health interviews.

2.7.1 Obesity rates among adults, 2007 (or latest year available)

2.7.2 Obesity rates among females and males, 2007 (or latest year available)

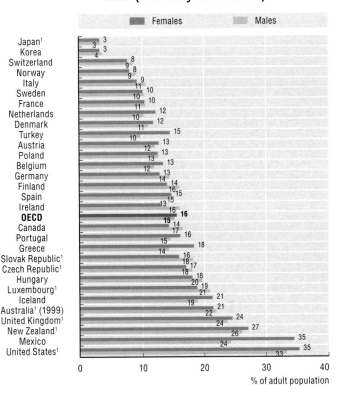

Country	2.7.1	Females	Males
Japan[1]	3.4	3	3
Korea	3.5	3	4
Switzerland	8.1	8	8
Norway	9.0	9	8
Italy	9.9	9	11
Sweden	10.2	10	10
France	10.5	10	10
Netherlands	11.2	11	12
Denmark	11.4	10	12
Turkey	12.0	11	15
Austria	12.4	10	13
Poland	12.5	12	13
Belgium	12.7	13	13
Germany	13.6	12	13
Finland	14.9	14	16
Spain	14.9	16	15
Ireland	15.0	15	13
OECD	**15.4**	16	**16**
Canada	15.4	15	14
Portugal	15.4	17	16
Greece	16.4	15	18
Slovak Republic[1]	16.7	14	16
Czech Republic[1]	17.0	18	17
Hungary	18.8	18	18
Luxembourg[1]	20.0	20	19
Iceland	20.1	21	21
Australia[1] (1999)	21.7	19	21
United Kingdom[1]	24.0	22	24
New Zealand[1]	26.5	24	27
Mexico	30.0	26	35
United States[1]	34.3	24	35
	33		

% of adult population

% of adult population

2.7.3 Increasing obesity rates among adults in OECD countries

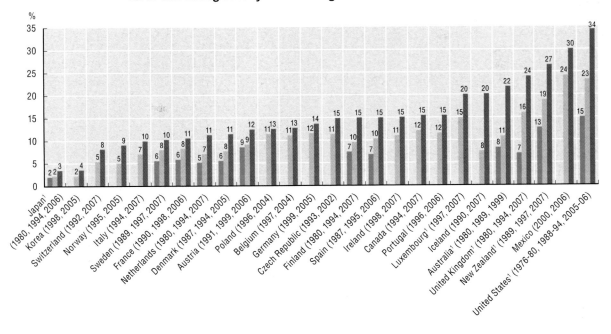

1. Australia, Czech Republic (2005), Japan, Luxembourg, New Zealand, Slovak Republic (2007), United Kingdom and United States figures are based on health examination surveys, rather than health interview surveys.

Source: OECD Health Data 2009.

StatLink ⓘ *http://dx.doi.org/10.1787/717854424544*

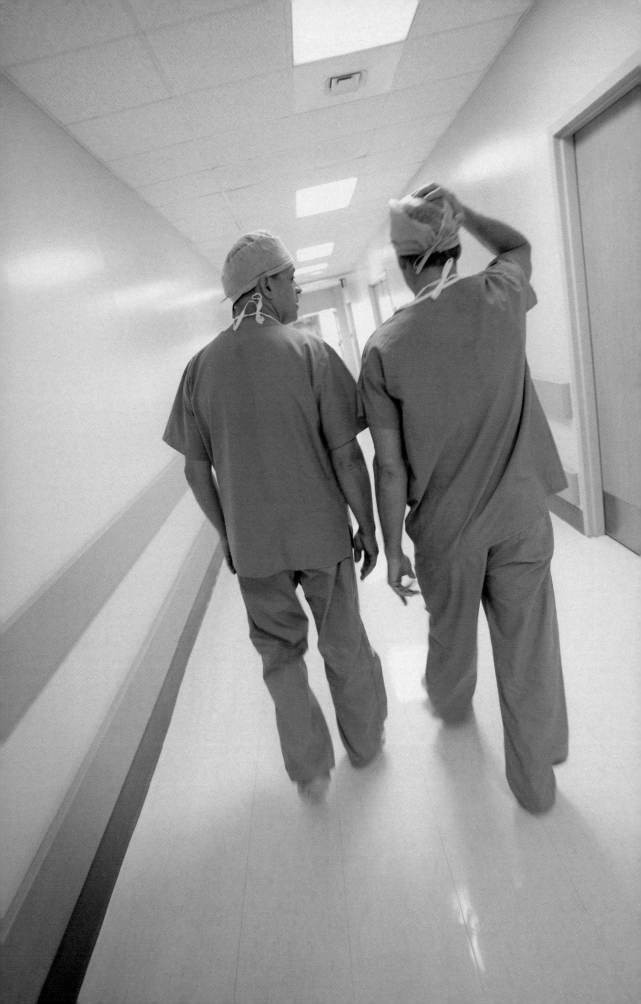

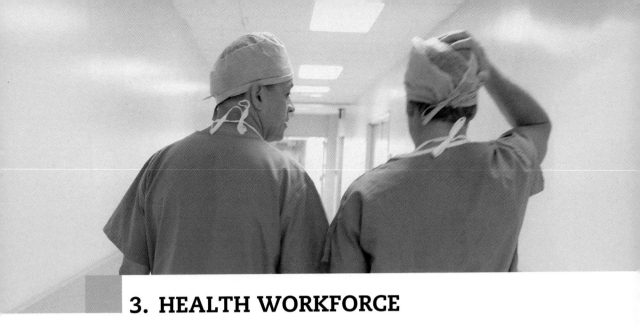

3. HEALTH WORKFORCE

Introduction

The performance of health systems in terms of access and quality depends crucially on the size, composition, distribution and productivity of the health workforce. Health workers are the cornerstone of health systems, and many OECD countries are reviewing their health human resource strategies to ensure a sufficient number of health care providers, with the right skills and in the right settings, to respond to the demand for high-quality health services.

This chapter provides the most recent data on the supply of health workers in OECD countries, along with some of the factors affecting the size and composition of the health workforce. It begins by providing a general overview of trends in employment in the health and social sectors, showing that these sectors account for a growing share of total employment in nearly all OECD countries. The rest of the chapter looks more specifically at certain health professions, with a particular focus on doctors and nurses.

The number of people working in the health sector is affected by inflows, which depend mainly on the entry of new graduates in the workforce and the immigration of foreign-trained workers, and by outflows, including retirement, emigration to other countries and temporary or permanent exits from the profession (Figure 3.1).

3.1 Supply of health workers: inflows, stocks and outflows

Source: OECD (2008e).

The two main methods of increasing the supply of doctors, nurses and other health professionals, as shown in Figure 3.1, are to increase domestic training or to recruit them abroad. These two methods have, however, quite different characteristics in terms of dynamics and impacts because of the long education and training periods, particularly for doctors. While foreign-trained doctors may be able to respond relatively quickly to any current shortages, it may take about ten years between any policy decision to increase the supply of new doctors and the time that they enter the workforce.

This chapter shows that there are large variations in the number of practising physicians and nurses across OECD countries. It also presents trends in the number of new graduates from medical and nursing education programmes as a key determinant of current and future supply, as well as trends in the number of foreign-trained doctors in OECD countries.*

Remuneration levels are one of the factors influencing the attractiveness of health professions, retention rates, and the possible migration of workers to other countries. The income levels of health workers also have a direct impact on the overall cost of health systems, since they represent a major expenditure item. Although it is difficult to gather comparable data on the remuneration of different categories of doctors and nurses, the evidence presented in this chapter suggests that there are large variations across countries, either in terms of absolute income levels across countries or compared to the average wage in each country. For doctors, differences in income levels can be attributed partly to the use of different remuneration methods (such as salary, capitation, or fee-for-services), and their impact on activity rates. However, differences in remuneration methods and activity rates do not explain all of the variations in remuneration levels, suggesting that the income of doctors are also affected by the prices (fees or salaries) that are negotiated for their services.

This chapter also provides information on the composition of the medical and nursing workforce. It shows that there is a growing imbalance between general practitioners and specialists in many OECD countries, raising issues about access to primary care. It also looks at the supply of certain categories of specialists, such as gynaecologists and obstetricians, and psychiatrists, taking advantage of the recent extension of the OECD data collection to these specialties. Many OECD countries are reporting shortages of GPs and specialists in certain regions, typically in rural and remote areas. Chapter 6 on "Access to care" provides some information on the uneven distribution of doctors within countries.

Two broad categories of nurses are distinguished in this chapter, "professional nurses" and "associate professional nurses" (who may be designated by different names in different countries). However, nursing aids, whom in some countries represent a very large group of care providers, are not included in the profile of nurse-related workers. This gap shows that information on the health care workforce continues to be limited in many areas.

---

* Data on the number of foreign-trained nurses around the year 2000 were reported in the 2007 edition of the OECD's *International Migration Outlook* (see Part III, "Immigrant Health Workers in OECD Countries in the Broader Context of Highly-Skilled Migration").

3. HEALTH WORKFORCE

3.1. Employment in the health and social sectors

The health and social sectors employ a large and growing number of people in OECD countries. The data reported in this section include people working in the health sector along with those working in the social sector (including long-term care, child care and other types of social work). The data include professionals providing direct services to people together with administrative and other support staff.

On average across OECD countries, employment in the health and social sectors accounted for nearly 10% of total employment in 2008, up from less than 9% in 1995. The share of people working in the health and social sectors in 2008 is highest in Nordic countries and the Netherlands, accounting for 15% or more of total employment. It is the lowest in Turkey and Mexico at about 3% (Figure 3.1.1).

The share of people employed in the health and social sectors has increased in nearly all OECD countries between 1995 and 2008, with the exception of Poland where it declined between 2000 and 2003 at a time of slow growth in health spending. In Iceland, Sweden and the Slovak Republic, the share has remained stable.

Between 1995 and 2008, the workforce in the health and social sectors grew by 2.8% per year on average across OECD countries, two-times faster than the growth rate of 1.4% in total civilian employment (Figure 3.1.2). In Korea, the number of people working in the health and social sectors increased at an average rate of over 8% per year during that period, compared with a growth rate in total employment of 1.1%. Nonetheless, the share of employment in the health and social sectors in Korea remains low compared with most other OECD countries. In Japan, the employment growth rate in the health and social sectors has also exceeded by a wide margin the growth rate in total employment in recent years.

In most countries, employment in the health and social sectors continued to increase between 2007 and 2008, at a time when total civilian employment started to

decline in some countries as their economy entered into recession. This was the case, for instance, in Japan, Spain and the United States, indicating that employment in the health and social sector was less affected by the economic downturn in these countries. However, in other countries such as the Czech Republic, Hungary and the Slovak Republic, employment in the health and social sectors fell between 2007 and 2008.

The majority of workers in the health sector are health professionals providing direct services to patients. The following indicators provide more detailed information on key health professions, including different categories of doctors and nurses, dentists and pharmacists.

3.1.1 Employment in the health and social sectors as a share of total civilian employment, 1995 and 2008 (or nearest year available)

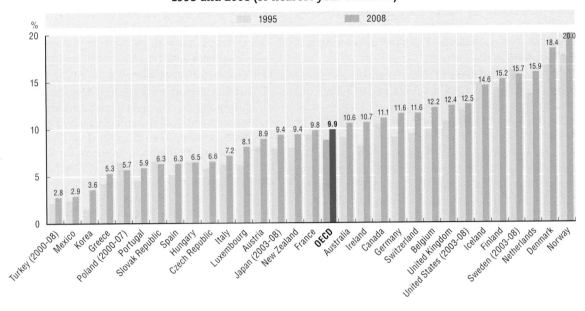

3.1.2 Employment growth rate in the health and social sectors compared with all sectors in the economy, 1995 to 2008 (or nearest year available)

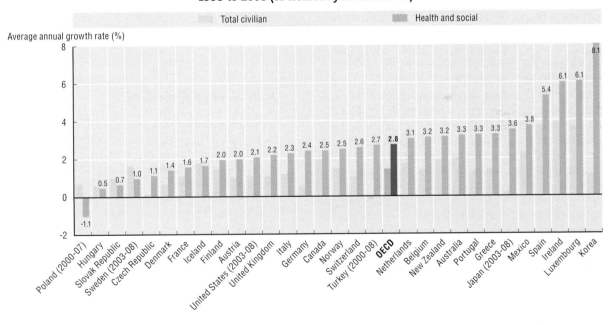

Source: OECD Annual Labour Force Statistics; US Bureau of Labor Statistics.

StatLink ⬛⬛ http://dx.doi.org/10.1787/717861583683

3. HEALTH WORKFORCE

3.2. Practising physicians

In many OECD countries, there are concerns about current or looming shortages of doctors (OECD, 2008e). This section provides information on the number of doctors per capita in OECD countries, including a disaggregation by gender and by general practitioners and specialists.

In 2007, there were highs of four practising doctors or more per 1 000 population in Greece and Belgium, and lows of less than two per 1 000 in Turkey and Korea (Figure 3.2.1). The OECD average was 3.1 per 1 000 population.

The ratio of practising physicians per 1 000 population has grown since 1990 in nearly all OECD countries. On average across OECD countries, physician density grew at a rate of 2% per year between 1990 and 2007 (Figure 3.2.2). The growth rate was particularly rapid in countries which started with lower levels in 1990 (Turkey, Korea and Mexico) as well as in Spain (since 1995) and Austria. In Austria, graduation rates from medical education programmes have consistently been above the OECD average during that period, resulting in high and rising numbers of doctors. On the other hand, the growth rate in the number of physicians per capita was much slower in Canada and France, and it was even negative in Italy. Following the reduction in the number of new entrants in medical schools during the 1980s and 1990s based on the view that there were too many physicians, the number of doctors per capita began to decline in Italy from 2003 and from 2006 in France. This downward trend is expected to continue.

In 2007, 40% of doctors on average across OECD countries were women, up from 29% in 1990 (Figure 3.2.3), ranging from highs of more than half in central and eastern European countries (Slovak Republic, Poland, Czech Republic and Hungary) and Finland to lows of less than 20% in Japan. In the United States, the proportion of female doctors has increased from 20% to 30% between 1990 and 2007, and it should continue to increase in the years ahead, as women enrolled in medical schools now account for nearly half of all students (NCHS, 2009).

The balance between general practitioners and specialists has changed over the past few decades, with the number of specialists increasing much more rapidly than generalists. Although health policy and health research tend to emphasise the importance and cost-effectiveness of generalist primary care (Starfield *et al.*, 2005), on average across OECD countries, there are now two specialists for every GP. This ratio was one-and-a-half in 1990. Specialists greatly outnumber generalists

in central and eastern European countries and in Greece. On the other hand, some countries have maintained a more equal balance between specialists and generalists (Australia, Belgium, Canada, France, New Zealand and Portugal), although even in some of these countries a vast majority of medical students are now choosing to specialise.

Forecasting the future supply and demand of doctors is difficult, because of uncertainties concerning overall economic growth, changes in physician productivity, advances in medical technologies, and the changing roles of physicians *versus* other care providers. In the United States, the Association of American Medical Colleges has estimated that the *demand* for physicians might increase by 26% between 2006 and 2025, while the *supply* might only increase by 10-12%, leading to a growing shortage of physicians (AAMC, 2008). In France, recent projections from the French Ministry of Health indicate that the *supply* of doctors may decline by almost 10% between 2006 and 2020, even taking into account the possible increase in the student intake from 7 000 places in 2006 to 8 000 places from 2011 to 2020 (DREES, 2009). Considering the growth in population during that period, the doctor-to-population ratio in France is expected to decline sharply, to reach a level of less than 2.8 doctors per 1 000 population in 2020, down from 3.35 in 2007, a decline of over 15% (DREES, 2009).

Definition and deviations

Practising physicians are defined as the number of doctors who are providing care directly to patients. In many countries, the numbers include interns and residents (doctors in training). The numbers are based on head counts, except in Norway which reported full-time equivalents prior to 2002. Ireland, the Netherlands, New Zealand and Portugal report the number of physicians entitled to practice (resulting in an over-estimation). Data for Spain include dentists and stomatologists (also resulting in a slight over-estimation).

Not all countries are able to report all their practising physicians in the two broad categories of specialists and generalists. This may be due to the fact that specialty-specific data are not available for doctors in training or for those working in private practice.

3.2.1 Practising physicians per 1 000 population, 2007 (or latest year available)

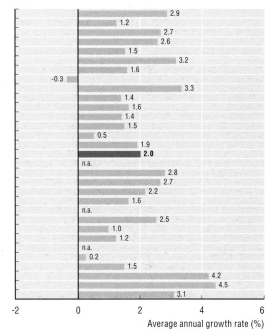

Country	Per 1 000 population
Greece	5.4
Belgium	4.0
Netherlands[1]	3.9
Norway	3.9
Switzerland	3.9
Austria	3.8
Iceland	3.7
Italy	3.7
Spain[2]	3.7
Sweden	3.6
Czech Republic	3.6
Portugal[1]	3.5
Germany	3.5
France	3.4
Denmark	3.2
OECD	**3.1**
Slovak Republic	3.1
Ireland[1]	3.0
Finland	3.0
Luxembourg	2.9
Australia	2.8
Hungary	2.8
United Kingdom	2.5
United States	2.4
New Zealand[1]	2.3
Poland	2.2
Canada	2.2
Japan	2.1
Mexico	2.0
Korea	1.7
Turkey	1.5

3.2.2 Growth in practising physician density, 1990-2007 (or nearest year)

Country	Average annual growth rate (%)
Greece	2.9
Belgium	1.2
Netherlands[1]	2.7
Norway	2.6
Switzerland	1.5
Austria	3.2
Iceland	1.6
Italy	-0.3
Spain[2]	3.3
Sweden	1.4
Czech Republic	1.6
Portugal[1]	1.4
Germany	1.5
France	0.5
Denmark	1.9
OECD	**2.0**
Slovak Republic	n.a.
Ireland[1]	2.8
Finland	2.7
Luxembourg	2.2
Australia	1.6
Hungary	n.a.
United Kingdom	2.5
United States	1.0
New Zealand[1]	1.2
Poland	n.a.
Canada	0.2
Japan	1.5
Mexico	4.2
Korea	4.5
Turkey	3.1

1. Ireland, the Netherlands, New Zealand and Portugal provide the number of all physicians entitled to practise rather than only those practising.   2. Data for Spain include dentists and stomatologists.

3.2.3 Female physicians as a percentage of all physicians, 1990 and 2007 (or nearest year)

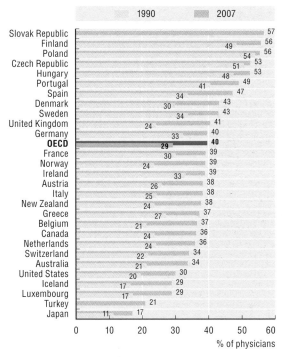

Country	1990	2007
Slovak Republic		57
Finland	49	56
Poland		56
Czech Republic	54	53
Hungary	51	53
Portugal	48	49
Spain	41	47
Denmark	34	43
Sweden	30	43
United Kingdom	34	41
Germany	24	40
OECD	**29**	**40**
France	33	39
Norway	30	39
Ireland	24	39
Austria	33	38
Italy	26	38
New Zealand	25	38
Greece	24	37
Belgium	27	37
Canada	21	36
Netherlands	24	36
Switzerland	24	34
Australia	22	34
United States	21	30
Iceland	20	29
Luxembourg	17	29
Turkey	17	21
Japan	11	17

3.2.4 General practitioners and specialists per 1 000 population, 2007 (or latest year available)

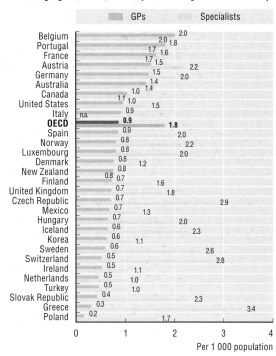

Country	GPs	Specialists
Belgium	2.0	1.8
Portugal	1.7	1.6
France	1.7	1.5
Austria	1.5	2.2
Germany	1.5	2.0
Australia	1.4	1.4
Canada	1.0	1.0
United States	1.1	1.5
Italy	0.9	n.a.
OECD	**0.9**	**1.8**
Spain	0.9	2.0
Norway	0.8	2.2
Luxembourg	0.8	2.0
Denmark	0.8	1.2
New Zealand	0.8	
Finland	0.7	1.6
United Kingdom	0.7	1.8
Czech Republic	0.7	2.9
Mexico	0.7	1.3
Hungary	0.6	2.0
Iceland	0.6	2.3
Korea	0.6	1.1
Sweden	0.5	2.6
Switzerland	0.5	2.8
Ireland	0.5	1.1
Netherlands	0.5	1.0
Turkey	0.5	1.0
Slovak Republic	0.4	2.3
Greece	0.3	3.4
Poland	0.2	1.7

Note: Some countries are unable to report all their practising doctors in these two categories of GPs and specialists.

Source: OECD Health Data 2009.

StatLink ⊞⊡⊑ http://dx.doi.org/10.1787/717877483033

3.3. Medical graduates

Maintaining or increasing the number of doctors requires either investment in training new doctors or recruiting trained physicians from abroad (see Indicator 3.4 "Foreign-trained physicians"). If it takes about ten years to train a doctor, any current shortages can be met only by recruiting qualified doctors from abroad, unless there are unemployed doctors at home. Conversely, any surpluses or sudden fall in demand may mean that new graduates, in particular, struggle to find vacant posts at home.

Virtually all OECD countries exercise some form of control over medical school intakes, often in the form of a *numerus clausus*. Such control is motivated by different factors including: i) confining medical entry to the most able applicants; ii) the desire to control the total number of doctors for cost-containment reasons (because greater supply induces greater demand); and iii) the cost of training itself (in all countries, including the United States, a significant part of medical education costs are publicly funded, so expansion of the number of medical students involves significant public expenditure). A *numerus clausus* is a policy instrument which countries have used by changing the cap at different times (OECD, 2008e).

Denmark, Austria and Ireland had, in 2007, the highest number of medical graduates per 100 000 population. These countries also tend to have more relaxed policies concerning medical student intakes. On the other hand, the graduation rates were the lowest in France, Japan, Canada and the United States. The average across OECD countries was close to ten new medical graduates per 100 000 population (Figure 3.3.1).

Measured in proportion to the stock of physicians (*i.e.* a measure of the replacement rate), the number of new medical graduates in 2007 was also the highest in Denmark, Austria and Ireland, along with Korea (which still has a relatively low number of doctors per capita). It was the lowest in France, Belgium and Switzerland. The average across OECD countries was 33 medical graduates per 1 000 practising doctors (Figure 3.3.2).

In several countries (*e.g.* Canada, Denmark and the United Kingdom), the number of medical graduates has started to rise strongly since 2000, following stable or declining graduation numbers in the preceding fifteen years, reflecting deliberate changes in policies to train more doctors (Figure 3.3.3). In Japan, the number of medical graduates has remained more or less unchanged over the past two decades. In Italy, France and Germany, there was a marked decline in the number of medical graduates between the

mid-1980s and the mid-1990s, after which it either continued to fall but a slower rate in the case of France and Germany (with a sign of a possible trend reversal in Germany in 2007) or to generally stabilised in the case of Italy.

In France, the *numerus clausus* was set at a high level (above 8 000 students) when it was first introduced in 1971, but it declined sharply in the late 1970s and 1980s to reach a low of 3 500 in 1992. It then rose to 7 100 by 2007, and consultations are underway to further increase it by 2012. However, given the time it takes to train new doctors, this recent increase in medical school intakes is not expected to be sufficient to maintain the number of doctors per capita in France in the coming years, as most doctors are now over 50 years old and expected to retire over the next decade (Cash and Ulmann, 2008).

In Japan, which has one of the lowest physician densities in the OECD area, doctor shortages have been discussed for some years and attributed to limits on the number of medical students (Ebihara, 2007). An Advisory Committee to the Japanese Ministry of Health, Labour and Welfare recently recommended an increase in the country's capacity to train new doctors by 50%, with the aim of increasing the number of doctors per capita from two per 1 000 population to the OECD average of three per 1 000. The intake of medical students has been increased since 2008, but it will take a long time to reach such a target.

Definition and deviations

Medical graduates are defined as the number of students who have graduated from medical schools or similar institutions in a given year. Dental, public health and epidemiology graduates are excluded.

The Czech Republic and the United Kingdom exclude foreign graduates, while other countries include them (foreign graduates account for about 30% of all medical graduates in the Czech Republic). In Denmark, the data refer to the number of new doctors receiving an authorization to practice.

In Luxembourg, the university does not provide medical training, so all doctors are foreign-trained, most of them in Belgium, France and Germany.

3.3.1 Medical graduates per 100 000 population, 2007 (or latest year available)

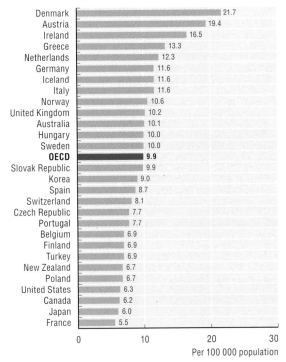

Per 100 000 population

3.3.2 Medical graduates per 1 000 practising physicians, 2007 (or latest year available)

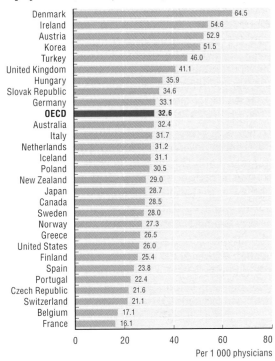

Per 1 000 physicians

3.3.3 Absolute number of medical graduates, selected OECD countries, 1985 to 2007

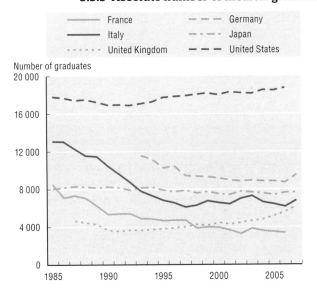

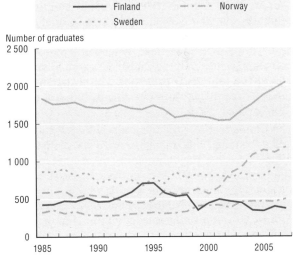

Source: OECD Health Data 2009.

StatLink ⌐⌐⌐ http://dx.doi.org/10.1787/718026057461

The international migration of doctors has raised a lot of attention among policy makers during the past decade. In 2007, the percentage of foreign-trained doctors ranges from a low of 3.1% in France (although this figure is under-estimated; see "Definition and deviations" below) to a high of 33.6% in Ireland (Figure 3.4.1). High percentages are also recorded in New Zealand and the United Kingdom where almost a third of all doctors were trained abroad. In Australia and the United States, this percentage is respectively 22.8% (2006) and 25.9%.

Differences across countries reflect, to a large extent, differences in migration patterns in general and the migration of highly-skilled workers in particular. The United Kingdom and New Zealand are, however, outliers as in these two countries the share of foreign-born among all tertiary educated workers is much lower than for physicians (OECD, 2008e).

The migration of doctors has risen over the past few years in many OECD countries. Changes in immigration policies and the development of bridging programmes for the recognition of foreign qualifications have contributed to this rise, but recent international recruitments have mainly been driven by unmet needs in host countries. Recent shortages of doctors are due to stringent measures on medical education adopted by many OECD countries over the past decades (see Indicator 3.3). Recent efforts to train more doctors should help reverse this trend, although the impact may only be felt in a few years.

The percentage of foreign-trained physicians has increased in most OECD countries, sometimes dramatically (Figure 3.4.2). It has nearly doubled in Switzerland and tripled in Ireland between 2000 and 2007. The increase also exceeded 5 percentage points in Sweden and the United Kingdom. Canada is one of the few OECD countries where the share of foreign-trained doctors has decreased since 2000 (Dumont et al., 2008).

The United States is the main receiving country, and hosts about half of all foreign-trained doctors working in the OECD. It is the only country to be a net receiver vis-à-vis all other OECD countries. In general, the international migration of health workers involves multiple interactions between OECD countries. Almost 60% of all migrant doctors in New Zealand were trained in another OECD country. This figure was 27% in the United Kingdom, 28% in the United States, 42% in Canada, and 90% in the Netherlands.

The composition of migration flows by country of origin depends on a number of factors, including: i) the importance of migratory ties; ii) language; and iii) recognition of qualifications. Figure 3.4.3 provides an illustration of the distribution of the countries of training for the two main OECD receiving countries, the United States and the United Kingdom. It confirms the importance of other OECD countries, but also points out the importance of inflows from large developing countries, notably India and the Philippines.

Even if smaller countries lose a small number of doctors in absolute term, this may have a large impact on their health system. Previous OECD work has shown, however, that the needs for health workers in developing countries, as estimated by the WHO, largely outstrip the numbers of immigrant health workers in the OECD (OECD, 2007a). Thus, it appears that international migration is neither the main cause nor would its reduction be the solution to the worldwide health human resources crisis, although it exacerbates the problem in some countries. There is growing awareness that the health workforce crisis is a global issue and that developing and developed countries need to work together to address it (OECD and WHO, 2009).

Definition and deviations

The data relate to registered foreign-trained physicians. In some countries however, the only information available relates to foreign doctors (without information on the location of their training). Some countries only report doctors with full registration, while others also include those with conditional/temporary/restrictive permits. Because migrant doctors are often over-represented in the latter categories, this may result in a serious undercounting of the number of foreign-trained doctors in those countries where they are not included. This is the case notably for France and to a lesser extent Ireland and Finland.

In most countries, the percentage of foreign-trained doctors is calculated by dividing it by the number of registered doctors. This is not the case, however, for France, Switzerland and the United Kingdom, where the share is calculated based on the number of practising doctors.

3.4.1 Share of foreign-trained or foreign doctors, 2007 (or latest year available)

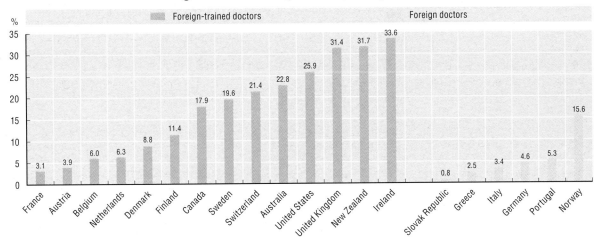

Source: OECD Health Data 2009 for foreign-trained doctors; OECD International Migration Outlook 2007 for foreign doctors.

3.4.2 Trends in the share of foreign-trained doctors, selected OECD countries, 2000-07

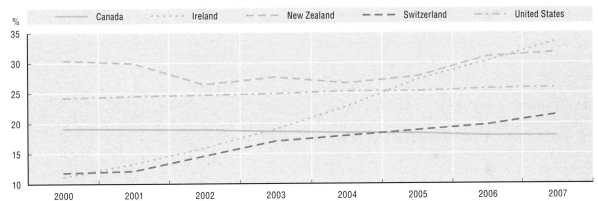

Source: OECD Health Data 2009.

3.4.3 Main countries of training of foreign-trained doctors, United States and United Kingdom

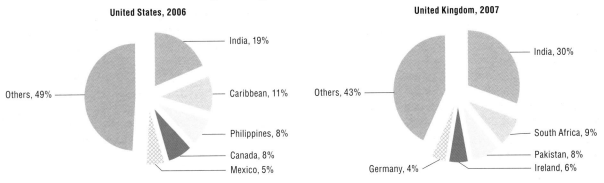

Source: OECD (www.oecd.org/health/workforce).

StatLink ᔕᔕᔐ *http://dx.doi.org/10.1787/718071211762*

Remuneration levels are among the factors affecting the attractiveness of different medical professions. They also affect health spending. Gathering comparable data on the remuneration of doctors is difficult, however, because countries collect data based on different sources covering different categories of physicians, and often not including all income sources (see the box on "Definition and deviations" below). Hence, the data should be interpreted with caution.

The data on the remuneration of doctors are presented for general practitioners (GPs) and specialists separately, comparing their remuneration with the average wage of all workers in each country. The remuneration of GPs ranges from 1.4 times the average wage of all workers in Hungary, to 4.2 times in the United Kingdom (Figure 3.5.1; right panel). The relative income of specialists ranges from 1.5 times the average wage of all workers for salaried specialists in Hungary, to 7.6 times for *self-employed* specialists in the Netherlands. The remuneration of *salaried* specialists in the Netherlands is lower, at 3.5 times the average wage (Figure 3.5.1; left panel). In the United States, the relative income of *self-employed* specialists was 5.6 times greater than the average wage in the country in 2001 (latest year available) and 4.1 times greater for *salaried* specialists.

In all countries, the remuneration of GPs is lower than that of specialists. The remuneration gap is particularly large in Australia, Belgium and the Netherlands, where GPs' earnings are less than half that of specialists. The gap is much smaller in Iceland and the United Kingdom.

In many countries, the remuneration of specialists has grown more quickly over the past five to ten years than that of GPs, widening the income gap (Figure 3.5.2). This has been the case in Australia, Finland, France and Hungary. In the United Kingdom, the incomes of both GPs and specialists have increased rapidly over the past ten years, with the growth rate in GP remuneration exceeding that of specialists. This can be attributed to the implementation of a new GP contract in 2004 designed to increase the number of GPs and improve the quality of primary care through better financial rewards. While the introduction of the new contract was expected to lead to additional cost, the actual cost in the first three years following its introduction was 9.4% higher than expected. There has been much debate in the United Kingdom on the gains that have been achieved in return for the extra spending (OECD, 2009d).

Some of the variations in the remuneration levels of GPs and specialists across countries can be explained by the use of different remuneration methods (*e.g.* salaries, fee-for-services, pay-for-performance schemes), by the role of GPs as gatekeepers, by differences in working time, and by the number of doctors per capita, particularly for specialists (Fujisawa and Lafortune, 2008).

3.5.1 Doctors' remuneration, ratio to average wage, 2007 (or latest year available)

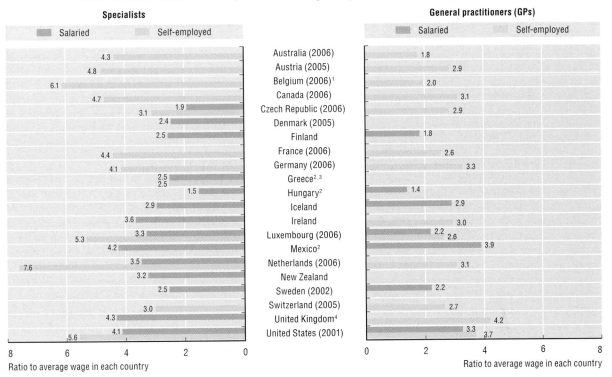

1. Data include practice expenses, resulting in an over-estimation.
2. Data on salaried doctors relate only to public sector employees who tend to receive lower remuneration than those working in the private sector.
3. Remuneration of salaried specialists is for 2005 and the income of self-employed specialists is for 2004.
4. Remuneration of self-employed GP is for 2006 and the income of salaried specialists is for 2007.

3.5.2 Growth in the remuneration of GPs and specialists

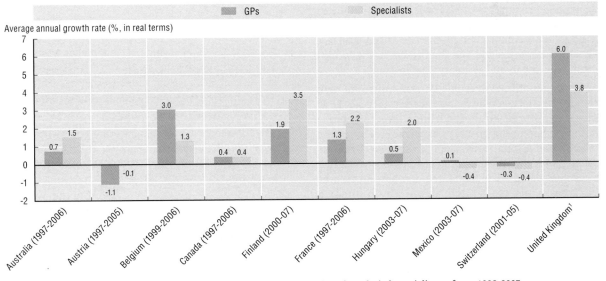

1. Data on remuneration for self-employed GPs refer to 1997-2006 and data for salaried specialists refer to 1998-2007.

Source: OECD Health Data 2009 for the remuneration of doctors; *OECD Employment Outlook 2009* and *OECD Taxing Wages 2009* for average wage of workers in the economy.

StatLink ᵐˢᵖ http://dx.doi.org/10.1787/718078600153

Gynaecologists are concerned with the functions and diseases specific to women, especially those affecting the reproductive system, while obstetricians specialise in pregnancy and childbirth. A doctor will often specialise in both these areas, and the data reported in this section does not allow a distinction between these two specialties. Midwives provide care and advice to women during pregnancy, labour and childbirth and the post-natal period for cases without complications. They deliver babies working independently or in collaboration with doctors and nurses.

In countries with a medicalised approach to pregnancy, obstetricians provide the majority of care. Where a less medicalised approach exists, trained midwives are the lead professionals, often working in collaboration with other health professionals like general practitioners, although obstetricians may be called upon if complications arise. Regardless of the different mix of providers across countries, the progress achieved over the past few decades in the provision of pre-natal advice and pregnancy surveillance, together with progress in obstetrics to deal with complicated births, have resulted in major reductions in perinatal mortality in all OECD countries.

The number of gynaecologists and obstetricians per 100 000 women is the highest in Greece, Czech Republic, Slovak Republic, Germany and Austria (Figure 3.6.1). These are all countries where obstetricians are given a primary role in providing pre-natal and childbirth care. It was the lowest in Ireland, the Netherlands, New Zealand and Canada.

Since 1995, the number of gynaecologists and obstetricians per woman has increased in most countries, with an average growth rate of just over 1% per year during that period. The number of gynaecologists and obstetricians per woman has remained relatively stable in Canada, France, Ireland and the United States, while it declined in Japan and Hungary (Figure 3.6.2).

The number of midwives per 100 000 women is highest in Australia, Iceland and Sweden (Figure 3.6.3). These two Nordic countries have a large number of midwives assuming primary responsibility for prenatal care and normal delivery (Johanson, 2002). On the other hand, the number of midwives per woman is the lowest in the United States, Canada and Korea. In Canada and the United States, the number of

midwives has increased at a rapid pace since 1995, but still remains very low compared with most other OECD countries (Figure 3.6.4). In Hungary, the number of midwives per woman has come down, with most of the reduction occurring between 2006 and 2007, as the number of beds in maternity wards was cut down by more than one-third in the context of a health reform. In the Czech Republic, the number of midwives per woman has also decreased, although part of the decline is due to a change in methodology in reporting midwives following the introduction of a new legislation in 2004.

The relative mix of providers has direct and indirect implications on the costs of pre-natal and natal services. Services involving midwives are likely to be cheaper. This reflects in part the lower training time and hence a lower required compensating pay for midwives in comparison to gynaecologists and obstetricians. Additionally, obstetricians may be inclined to provide more medicalised services. A study of nine European countries found that the cost of delivery is lower in those countries and hospitals that employ more midwives and nurses than obstetricians (Bellanger and Or, 2008).

There is little evidence that systems that rely more on midwives are less effective. A review of a number of studies finds that midwives are equally effective in providing pre-natal care and advice in the case of normal pregnancies (Di Mario et al., 2005), although support from obstetricians is required for complications. Some evidence from the United States suggests a better performance in term of neonatal mortality for midwife attended births (Miller, 2006).

Definition and deviations

The number of gynaecologists and obstetricians combines these two specialities.

The figures for gynaecologists and obstetricians, and for midwives, are presented in head counts, not taking into account how many of them may work full-time or part-time.

3.6.1 Gynaecologists and obstetricians per 100 000 females, 2007 (or latest year available)

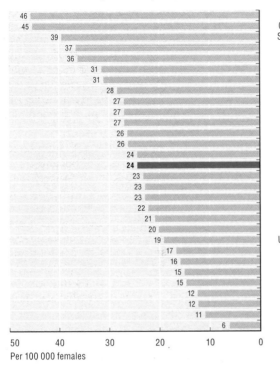

Per 100 000 females

3.6.2 Change in the number of gynaecologists and obstetricians per female, 1995-2007 (or nearest year)

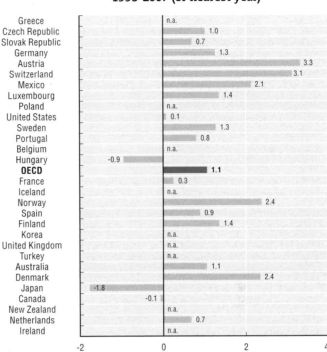

Average annual growth rate (%)

3.6.3 Midwives per 100 000 females, 2007 (or latest year available)

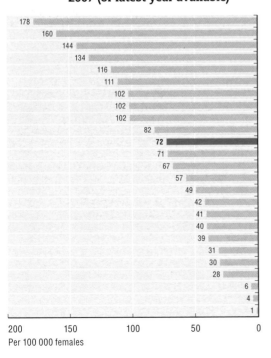

Per 100 000 females

3.6.4 Change in the number of midwives per female, 1995-2007 (or nearest year)

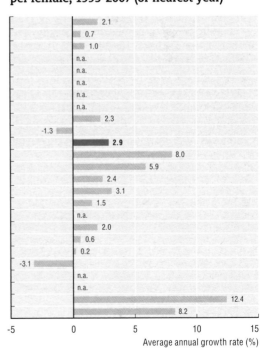

Average annual growth rate (%)

Source: OECD Health Data 2009.

StatLink http://dx.doi.org/10.1787/718151264476

At any point in time, about 10% of the adult population will report having some type of mental or behavioural disorder (WHO, 2001). People with mental health problems may receive help from a variety of professionals, including general practitioners, psychiatrists, psychologists, psychotherapists, social workers, specialist nurses and others. In Europe, a population-based survey carried out in 2005-06 indicated that, on average across EU countries, 13% of the population reported seeking help from a health professional for a psychological or emotional health problem over the past year (*Eurobarometer*, 2006). Among the people who sought help, two-thirds (67%) had consulted a general practitioner, while 15% sought help from a psychiatrist and another 15% from a psychologist (Figure 3.7.3).

This section focuses on one category of mental health service provider, psychiatrists, as the availability of comparable data on others, such as psychologists, is more limited. Psychiatrists are responsible for diagnosing and treating a variety of serious mental health problems, including depression, learning disabilities, alcoholism and drug addiction, eating disorders, and personality disorders such as schizophrenia. The number of psychiatrists in most OECD countries is between 10 and 20 per 100 000 population. The number is highest in Switzerland, some Nordic countries (Iceland and Norway) and France. It is the lowest in Turkey, Korea, Poland, Hungary and Spain (Figure 3.7.1).

The number of psychiatrists per capita has increased since 1995 in most OECD countries for which data are available. The rise has been particularly rapid in Luxembourg, Switzerland, Germany and Austria. On the other hand, there has been no increase in the number of psychiatrists per capita in France, Hungary, Portugal and the United States since 1995 (Figure 3.7.2). In France, most of the increase happened in the 1970s.

As is the case for many other medical specialties, psychiatrists may be unevenly distributed across regions within each country, with some regions being underserved. For example, in Australia, the number of psychiatrists per capita is seven times greater in major cities than in remote regions (AIHW, 2008b).

The role of psychiatrists varies across countries. A country like Spain has deliberately chosen to use psychiatrists to work in close co-operation with general practitioners (GPs). Hence, although the number of psychiatrists is relatively low, consultation rates of psychiatrists by people with mental disorders are higher than in other countries where the number of psychiatrists is higher, because of higher referral rates from their GPs (Kovess-Masfety, 2007).

The role of other mental health service providers such as psychologists also varies across countries. For instance, in the Netherlands, there is a high number of psychologists who are very active in providing services that are covered under health insurance systems. In other countries such as France, the number of psychologists is lower and the services that they provide are not covered under public health insurance (Kovess-Masfety, 2007).

Definition and deviations

Psychiatrists are medical doctors who specialize in the prevention, diagnosis and treatment of mental illness. They have post-graduate training in psychiatry, and may also have additional training in a psychiatric specialty, such as neuropsychiatry and child psychiatry. Psychiatrists can prescribe medication, which psychologists cannot do in most countries.

The figures normally include psychiatrists, neuropsychiatrists and child psychiatrists. Psychologists are excluded. The numbers are presented as head counts, regardless of whether psychiatrists work full-time or part-time.

3.7.1 Psychiatrists per 100 000 population, 2007 (or latest year available)

3.7.2 Change in the number of psychiatrists per 100 000 population, 1995-2007 (or nearest year)

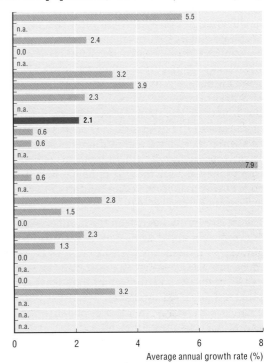

Country	Per 100 000 population	Average annual growth rate (%)
Switzerland	42	5.5
Iceland	26	n.a.
Norway	25	2.4
France	22	0.0
Belgium	20	n.a.
Austria	19	3.2
Germany	19	3.9
Sweden	18	2.3
United Kingdom	18	n.a.
OECD	**15**	**2.1**
Australia	15	0.6
Canada	15	0.6
Greece	15	n.a.
Luxembourg	15	7.9
Netherlands	15	0.6
New Zealand	15	n.a.
Czech Republic	14	2.8
Denmark	13	1.5
United States	13	0.0
Slovak Republic	11	2.3
Japan	10	1.3
Portugal	10	0.0
Ireland	9	n.a.
Hungary	8	0.0
Spain	8	3.2
Poland	6	n.a.
Korea	5	n.a.
Turkey	3	n.a.

Source: OECD Health Data 2009.

3.7.3 Type of provider(s) consulted for mental health problems, selected EU countries, 2005-06

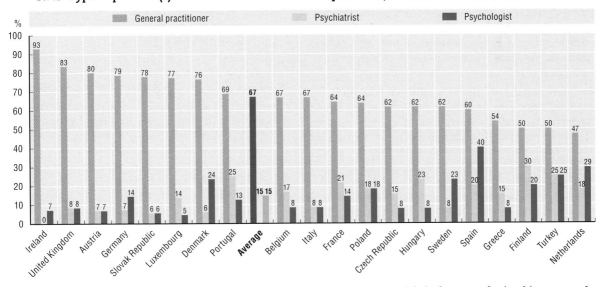

Note: The question asked during the interview was: "In the last 12 months, did you seek help from a professional in respect of a psychological or emotional health problem? If yes, indicate who in the provided list." Multiple answers were possible for the second part of the question.

Source: Eurobarometer, December 2005-January 2006.

StatLink ⊞⟋⟍ *http://dx.doi.org/10.1787/718154154448*

Nurses are usually the most numerous health profession, greatly outnumbering physicians in most OECD countries. Nurses play a critical role in providing health care not only in traditional settings such as hospitals and long-term care institutions but increasingly in primary care (especially in offering care to the chronically ill) and in domiciliary settings. However, there are concerns in many countries about shortages of nurses, and these concerns may well intensify in the future as the demand for nurses continues to increase and the ageing of the "baby boom" generation precipitates a wave of retirements among nurses. These concerns have prompted actions in many countries to increase the training of new nurses combined with efforts to increase the retention of nurses in the profession (OECD, 2008e).

This section presents data on the number of practising nurses, separating where applicable "professional nurses" from "associate professional nurses" (although these two categories of nurses often have different names in different countries). In 2007, there were over 30 nurses per 1 000 population in Norway, followed by Ireland with over 15, to a low of about two in Turkey and Mexico (Figure 3.8.1). The OECD average was 9.6 nurses per 1 000 population.

In Norway, more than half of nurses are "associate professionals" who have high-school education only and provide mainly social care. By contrast, in many other countries such as the United Kingdom and the United States, the vast majority of nurses are professional nurses. In some countries such as France, Portugal and Poland, the category of "associate professional nurses" does not exist, although professional nurses can be assisted by nursing aids who do not, however, have a formal recognition as a nurse.

The number of nurses per 1 000 population rose at an average rate of 1.4% per year between 2000 and 2007 across OECD countries (Figure 3.8.2). In Australia, the Netherlands and the Slovak Republic, the number of nurses per capita actually declined since 2000 (since 2004 in the case of the Netherlands). In Canada, following a decrease in the number of nurses per capita during the 1990s, the numbers have risen again over the past few years, following increased efforts to train more nurses (see Indicator 3.9 "Nursing graduates").

The United States has the largest nurse workforce of all OECD countries, with close to 3 million "professional nurses" and more than 700 000 "associate professional

nurses", but there is still a growing demand (Aiken and Cheung, 2008). Unless greater efforts are made to train more nurses, a shortage of one million professional nurses is projected in the United States by 2020 (HRSA, 2004). Some measures have already been taken to increase the number of graduates from nursing education programmes (see Indicator 3.9).

In 2007, the nurse-to-doctor ratio ranged from over five nurses per doctor in Norway and Ireland to under one nurse per doctor in Greece (Figure 3.8.3). The number of nurses per doctor is also relatively low in other southern European countries (Portugal, Italy and Spain). The average across OECD countries is just over three nurses per doctor, with most countries reporting between two to four nurses per doctor. In Greece and Italy, there is evidence of an over-supply of doctors and under-supply of nurses, resulting in an inefficient allocation of resources (OECD, 2009c; Chaloff, 2008).

Definition and deviations

Practising nurses include nurses employed in all public and private settings, including the self-employed, who are providing services directly to patients. In most countries, the data include both "professional nurses" who have a higher level of education and perform higher level tasks and "associate professional nurses" who have a lower level of education but are nonetheless recognised and registered as nurses. Midwives, nursing aids who are not recognised as nurses, and nurses working in administration and research should normally be excluded.

However, about half of OECD countries include midwives because they are considered as a specialist nurse, and a number of countries include non-practising nurses working in administration and research (resulting in an over-estimation). Austria reports only nurses working in hospitals, resulting in an under-estimation. Data for Germany does not include about 250 000 nurses (representing an additional 30% of nurses) who have three years of education and are providing services for the elderly.

3.8.1 Practising nurses per 1 000 population, 2007 (or latest year available)

3.8.2 Change in the number of practising nurses per 1 000 population, 2000-07

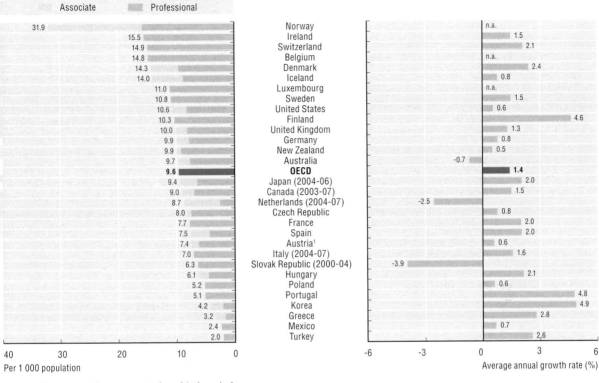

1. Austria reports only nurses employed in hospitals.

3.8.3 Ratio of practising nurses to practising physicians, 2007 (or latest year available)

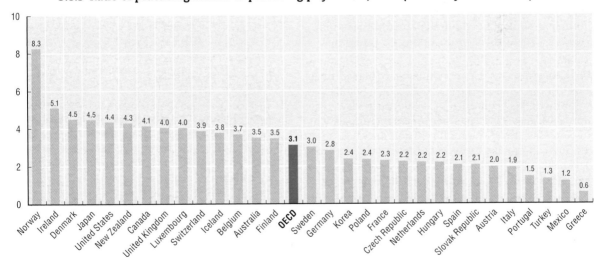

Source: OECD Health Data 2009.

StatLink 🔗 http://dx.doi.org/10.1787/718182651388

Many OECD countries have taken steps in recent years to expand the number of students in nursing education programmes in response to concerns about current or anticipated shortages of nurses. Increasing investment in nursing education is particularly important as the nursing workforce is ageing in many countries and the baby boom generation of nurses approaches retirement.

On average in OECD countries, there were 36 newly-graduated nurses per 100 000 population in 2007 (Figure 3.9.1). The number was the highest in the Slovak Republic, Norway and Switzerland. In the Slovak Republic, nurse graduation rates in 2007 were much higher than in preceding years, signalling recent efforts to increase the number of nurses. In Norway and Switzerland, nurse graduation rates have consistently been above the OECD average since the mid-1980s, explaining why these countries have a higher number of nurses per capita (see Indicator 3.8). On the other hand, nurse graduation rates have traditionally been low in Turkey, Greece and Italy, three countries which report a relatively low number of nurses per capita. In Luxembourg, nurse graduation rates are also low, but a large number of nurses are foreign-trained.

The institutional arrangements for nursing education differ across OECD countries. In some countries, the number of students admitted in nursing programmes is decided in a decentralised way, without any numerical limits. This is the case in Belgium, the Netherlands, Norway, New Zealand and the United States, although in this latter case State decisions on public funding for nursing education have a direct impact on the capacity of nursing schools to admit students. In most countries, however, entry into nursing programmes is regulated (OECD, 2008e).

When compared to the current number of nurses, there were 42 nurse graduates per 1 000 practising nurses on average in OECD countries in 2007 (Figure 3.9.2). The number of new graduates per practising nurses was high in the Slovak Republic, Korea and Portugal, although in the latter two countries this is partly explained by the relatively low number of nurses. The number of new graduates per practising nurses is the lowest in Luxembourg, which is compensated by the import of nurses trained in other countries. Nurse graduation rates are also low in Ireland which has also been relying on immigration to fill some of its need (OECD, 2007a).

In Italy, concerns about current and future shortages of nurses have led to a significant increase in student intake in university nursing programmes in recent years, resulting in a rise in the number of newly-graduated nurses from less than 6 000 in 2002 to over 10 000 in 2007. Nonetheless, this may not be sufficient to meet current and future demand, given that the number of nurses leaving the profession annually is estimated to be in the range of 13 000 to 17 000 (Chaloff, 2008).

In many OECD countries, there has been an increase in the number of students graduating from nursing programmes since 2000 (Figure 3.9.3). This has been the case, for instance, in France, Norway, Switzerland and the United States. In the United States, the Federal budget for fiscal year 2010 provides for additional funding to enhance the capacity of nursing schools to increase the number of nurses (Office of Management and Budget, 2009).

In Denmark, the number of nursing graduates has been relatively stable between 2000 and 2007, but the capacity of nursing colleges has also been increased by 10% since 2007 in response to reported shortages of nurses (OECD, 2008b). In Japan, the number of nursing graduates has declined between 2000 and 2007, reflecting a reduction in the number of nursing schools and student capacity. However, this reduction in training capacity has been reversed since 2006, which should lead to a growing number of graduates in the years ahead (Japanese Nursing Association, 2009).

Definition and deviations

Nursing graduates refer to the number of students who have obtained a recognised qualification required to become a licensed or registered nurse. They exclude graduates from Masters or PhD degrees in nursing to avoid double-counting people acquiring further qualifications.

The numbers reported by Canada, Iceland, New Zealand, Spain and the United States do not include graduates from lower level nursing programmes, nor are graduates from three-year education programmes focusing on elderly care included in Germany, resulting in an underestimation in graduation rates per capita. However, the calculation of graduation rates per practising nurses includes the same categories of nurses in the numerator and the denominator to avoid any under-estimation.

The United Kingdom excludes nursing graduates from overseas.

3.9.1 Nursing graduates per 100 000 population, 2007 (or latest year available)

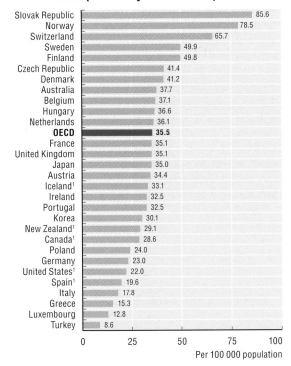

Per 100 000 population

3.9.2 Nursing graduates per 1 000 nurses, 2007 (or latest year available)

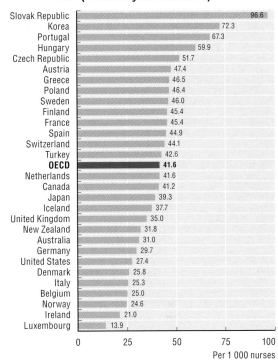

Per 1 000 nurses

1. The number of graduates reported by Canada, Iceland, New Zealand, Spain and the United States does not include graduates from lower level nursing programmes, resulting in an under-estimation compared with other countries in graduation rates per capita (Figure 3.9.1). However, the calculation of graduation rates per practising nurses (Figure 3.9.2) only include professional nurses (higher level nurses), to avoid any under-estimation.

3.9.3 Absolute number of nursing graduates, selected OECD countries, 1990-2007

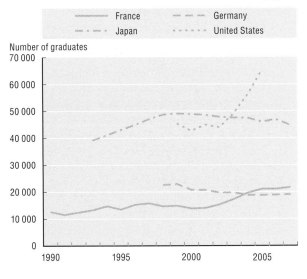

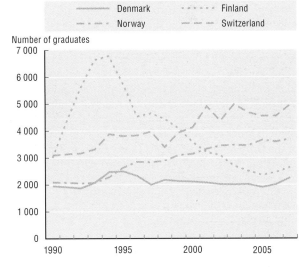

Source: OECD Health Data 2009.

StatLink http://dx.doi.org/10.1787/718187845226

The remuneration level of nurses is one of the factors affecting job satisfaction and the attractiveness of the profession. It also has a direct impact on costs, as wages represent one of the main spending items in health systems.

Gathering comparable data on the remuneration of nurses is difficult because different countries collect data based on different sources, covering different categories of nurses. The data presented in this section generally focus on the remuneration of nurses working in hospitals, although the data coverage for some countries differs (see the box below on "Definition and deviations"). Hence, the data should be interpreted with caution.

The data on the remuneration of nurses is presented in two ways. First, it is compared with the average wage of all workers in each country, providing some indication on the relative financial attractiveness of nursing compared to other occupations. Second, the remuneration level in each country is converted into a common currency, the US dollar, and adjusted for purchasing power parity, to provide an indication of the relative economic well-being of nurses compared with their counterparts in other countries.

In most countries, the remuneration of nurses is above the average wage of all workers in their country (Figure 3.10.1). This is particularly the case in Mexico, where the income of nurses is more than two times greater than the average wage. In Portugal, it is 70% higher. On the other hand, the income of nurses is lower than the average wage in Hungary, Slovak Republic, Czech Republic and Finland. In Finland, the growth in the salary of nurses lagged behind the growth in the average wage between 2000 and 2007, but in 2008, nurses have obtained a substantial pay raise which should narrow this gap.

When converted to a common currency, the remuneration of nurses is four to six times higher in Luxembourg than in Hungary, Slovak Republic and Czech Republic (Figure 3.10.2). Nurses in the United States also have relatively high earnings compared with their counterparts in other countries. This might explain the ability of the United States to attract many nurses from other countries (OECD, 2007a; Aiken and Cheung, 2008). In Mexico, although the salary of nurses appears to be high compared to other workers in the country, their income level is low compared to nurses in the United States and other countries.

The remuneration of nurses in real terms (taking into account inflation) has increased in all OECD countries over the past five to ten years, with the exception of Mexico where it declined between 2003 and 2007

(Figure 3.10.3). The growth rate in the remuneration of nurses was particularly strong in the Slovak Republic and the Czech Republic, narrowing the gap to a certain extent with their counterparts in other European countries. In the United Kingdom, the income of nurses in real terms grew at an average of 3% per year over the past ten years, two-times more rapidly than the growth in the average wage in the economy.

There is some evidence that low wage is one of the reasons why some nurses leave the profession (Hasselhorn et al., 2005). However, other research found only a weak relationship between wage and nurse labour supply (Shield, 2004; Chiha and Link, 2003; Antonazzo et al., 2003). Other policies, such as improving working-time flexibility and creating career development opportunities, may also help to attract and retain more nurses in the profession (OECD, 2008e).

Definition and deviations

The remuneration of nurses refers to average *gross* annual income, including social security contributions and income taxes payable by the employee. It should normally include all extra formal payments, such as bonuses and payments for night shifts and overtime. In most countries, the data relate specifically to nurses working in hospitals, although in New Zealand and the United States the data also cover nurses working in other settings.

Data refer only to registered ("professional") nurses in Australia, Denmark and Norway, resulting in an overestimation compared to other countries where lower-level nurses ("associate professional") are also included.

The data relate to nurses working full-time, with the exception of Belgium where part-time nurses are also included (resulting in an underestimation). The data for some countries do not include overtime payments (e.g. Ireland and Mexico). None of the countries report data on informal payments, which in some countries may represent a significant part of total income.

The remuneration of nurses is compared to the average wage of full-time employees in all sectors in the country, except in Iceland, Mexico and New Zealand where it is compared to the average wage in selected industrial sectors.

3.10.1 Hospital nurses' remuneration, ratio to average wage, 2007 (or latest year available)

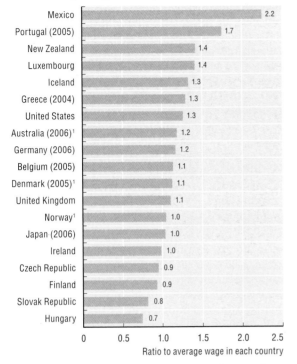

Ratio to average wage in each country

Country	Ratio
Mexico	2.2
Portugal (2005)	1.7
New Zealand	1.4
Luxembourg	1.4
Iceland	1.3
Greece (2004)	1.3
United States	1.3
Australia (2006)[1]	1.2
Germany (2006)	1.2
Belgium (2005)	1.1
Denmark (2005)[1]	1.1
United Kingdom	1.1
Norway[1]	1.0
Japan (2006)	1.0
Ireland	1.0
Czech Republic	0.9
Finland	0.9
Slovak Republic	0.8
Hungary	0.7

3.10.2 Hospital nurses' remuneration, USD PPP, 2007 (or latest year available)

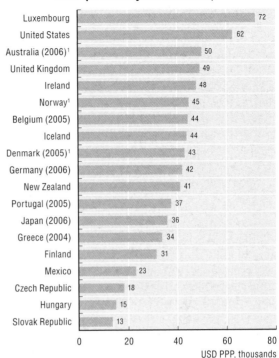

USD PPP, thousands

Country	USD PPP, thousands
Luxembourg	72
United States	62
Australia (2006)[1]	50
United Kingdom	49
Ireland	48
Norway[1]	45
Belgium (2005)	44
Iceland	44
Denmark (2005)[1]	43
Germany (2006)	42
New Zealand	41
Portugal (2005)	37
Japan (2006)	36
Greece (2004)	34
Finland	31
Mexico	23
Czech Republic	18
Hungary	15
Slovak Republic	13

1. Data refer to registered ("professional") nurses in Australia, Denmark and Norway.

3.10.3 Growth in the remuneration of hospital nurses

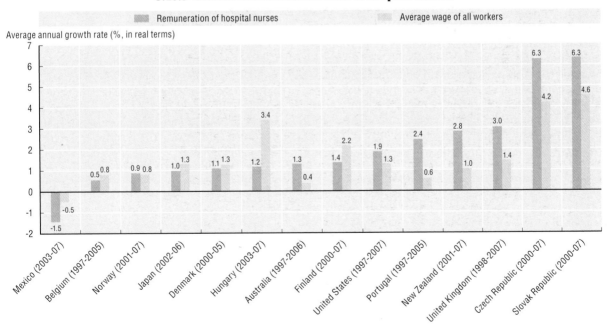

Remuneration of hospital nurses   Average wage of all workers

Average annual growth rate (%, in real terms)

Country	Remuneration of hospital nurses	Average wage of all workers
Mexico (2003-07)	-1.5	-0.5
Belgium (1997-2005)	0.5	0.8
Norway (2001-07)	0.9	0.8
Japan (2002-06)	1.0	1.3
Denmark (2000-05)	1.1	1.3
Hungary (2003-07)	1.2	3.4
Australia (1997-2006)	1.3	0.4
Finland (2000-07)	1.4	2.2
United States (1997-2007)	1.9	1.3
Portugal (1997-2005)	2.4	0.6
New Zealand (2001-07)	2.8	1.0
United Kingdom (1998-2007)	3.0	1.4
Czech Republic (2000-07)	6.3	4.2
Slovak Republic (2000-07)	6.3	4.6

Source: OECD Health Data 2009 for the remuneration of nurses; *OECD Employment Outlook 2009* and *OECD Taxing Wages 2009* for average wage of workers in the economy.

StatLink ᵐˢᵖ *http://dx.doi.org/10.1787/718276801843*

Dentists are the main provider of dental care, although some services are also provided by dental hygienists, dental assistants and dental prosthetists. Most dentists in OECD countries work in their own office or in a group practice (dental clinics), although a small proportion also work in hospitals and other health care facilities.

In most OECD countries, there are between 50 and 80 practising dentists per 100 000 population (Figure 3.11.1). Greece has the highest number of dentists per capita, followed by Iceland, Norway, Sweden, Belgium and Luxembourg, with 80 or more dentists per 100 000 population. The number of dentists per capita is the lowest in Mexico, although it has increased significantly since 1990.

Between 1990 and 2007, the number of dentists per capita has increased in nearly all OECD countries, except Finland, Sweden and Denmark where numbers were high to start with and remain well above the OECD average. The number of dentists per capita has risen particularly strongly in Portugal (it has more than tripled in absolute terms since 1990), and in Spain and Korea (the absolute number has more than doubled), although they remain well below the OECD average in Korea (Figure 3.11.2).

In countries such as France, the Netherlands and the United States, the number of dentists increased at the same pace as the growth in the population, resulting in a stable number of dentists per capita between 1990 and 2007.

A higher number of dentists per capita generally tends to be associated with a higher number of dentist consultations (Figure 3.11.3). However, for a given number of dentists per capita, there can still be wide differences in the average number of dentist consultations. For instance, while Japan has slightly fewer dentists per capita than Germany, Finland and Denmark, the average number of dentist consultations is two to three times greater.

Estimates of annual numbers of consultations per dentist can be derived by using information on dentist consultations. Caution should be used in interpreting this indicator as a measure of dentists' productivity, because consultations (which can include treatments) can vary in complexity, length and effectiveness. Nevertheless, Figure 3.11.4 shows large variations in the estimated number of consultations per dentist, with up to four-fold differences across OECD countries. This might be due partly to differences in average working hours and partly also to differences in the availability of support staff and assistants allowing dentists to see more patients per day. In Mexico, the significant increase in the number of dentists per capita since 1990 has been accompanied by relatively low activity rates, suggesting that the growth in supply may be exceeding the increase in the demand for dental care. By contrast, the strong increase in the supply of dentists in Korea since 1990 has been associated with high activity rates.

As is the case with other health professionals, there tends to be a higher number of dentists per capita in large cities than in rural areas. For instance, in France, there were four times more dentists per capita in Paris than in rural communities in 2006 (DREES, 2007). The low supply of dentists in rural areas might result in unmet dental care needs (see Indicator 6.1 "Unmet health care needs").

Definition and deviations

The number of dentists includes both salaried and self-employed dentists. In most countries, the data only include dentists providing direct services to clients/patients. This is not the case however in Canada, Ireland, Portugal and Spain, where the data relate to all dentists licensed to practice, including those who may not be actively practising.

3.11.1 Dentists per 100 000 population, 2007 (or latest year available)

3.11.2 Change in the number of dentists per 100 000 population, 1990-2007 (or nearest year)

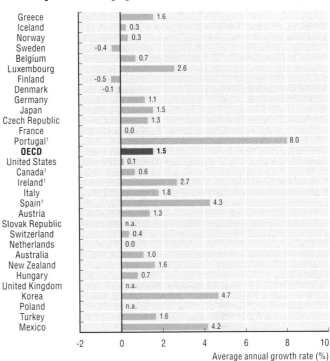

Per 100 000 population

Average annual growth rate (%)

1. Canada, Ireland, Portugal and Spain provide the number of all dentists licensed to practise rather than only those practising.

3.11.3 Number of dentists and dentist consultations per capita, 2007 (or latest year available)

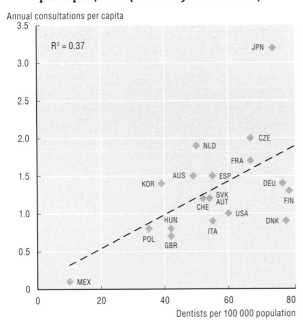

Annual consultations per capita

Dentists per 100 000 population

3.11.4 Estimated number of consultations per dentist, 2007 (or latest year available)

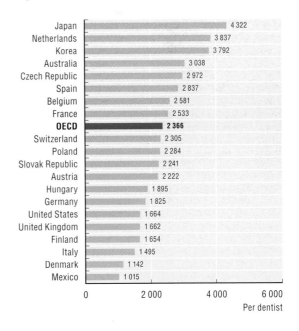

Per dentist

Source: OECD Health Data 2009.

StatLink 🖳🖧 *http://dx.doi.org/10.1787/718311135608*

Pharmacists assist people in obtaining medication and ensuring that these are used in a safe and proper fashion. In most countries, they have completed studies in pharmacy at university level and have completed an examination administered by the regulatory authority to obtain a license to practice.

In most OECD countries, there are between 60 and 100 pharmacists per 100 000 population. Japan, France and Belgium have the highest number of pharmacists per capita, with rates above 115 per 100 000 population (Figure 3.12.1). This high rate is associated with a high number of community pharmacies (Figure 3.12.3). On the other hand, the number of pharmacists per capita is the lowest in Denmark and the Netherlands, which is also related to the fact that these two countries have among the lowest number of community pharmacies per capita. The relatively low number of community pharmacies in the Netherlands may be explained partly by the fact that patients can also purchase their prescription drugs directly from some doctors who are dispensing medications (Vogler *et al.*, 2008).

Between 1990 and 2007, the number of pharmacists per capita has increased in nearly all OECD countries, with the exception of Denmark and Belgium, although it remains high in Belgium. It increased most rapidly in Spain, Japan, Ireland, Portugal and Hungary (Figure 3.12.2).

In Japan, the strong increase in the number of pharmacists can be attributed to a large extent to the government's efforts to separate more clearly drug prescribing by doctors from drug dispensing by pharmacists (the so-called *Bungyo* system). Traditionally, the vast majority of prescription drugs in Japan were dispensed directly by doctors. However, in recent years, the Japanese government has taken a number of steps to encourage the separation of drug prescribing from dispensing. In 1997, the Medical Service Law was amended to recognise the role of pharmacists as health professionals. The Medical Service Law was amended in 2006 and recognised community pharmacies as facilities providing health goods and services. Following these amendments, the percentage of prescriptions dispensed by pharmacists rose from 26% of all prescriptions in 1997 to 57% in 2007, while the number of community pharmacies increased from 42 412 to 52 539 (Japanese Pharmaceutical Association, 2008).

Most pharmacists work in community pharmacies. For instance, in Canada, 75% of all practising pharmacists work in community pharmacies, while 15% to 20% work in hospitals and other health care facilities, and the remaining 5% to 10% work in the industrial sector and other settings (CIHI, 2008b). In Japan, 50% of pharmacists worked in community pharmacies in 2006, up from one-third in 1990 (Japanese Pharmaceutical Association, 2008).

Definition and deviations

Practising pharmacists are defined as the number of pharmacists who are licensed to practice and provide direct services to clients/patients. They can be either salaried or self-employed, and work in community pharmacies, hospitals and other settings. Assistant pharmacists and other employees of pharmacies are normally excluded.

The data from the Netherlands exclude pharmacists working in hospitals/clinics (resulting in a slight under-estimation). The data for Luxembourg exclude pharmacists paid by hospitals, but include employees in pharmacies and pharmacists working in administration.

In Ireland, the data include all people on the register of the Pharmaceutical Society of Ireland, possibly including some pharmacists who are not in activity. In addition, the figures include assistant pharmacists, pharmaceutical assistants, and doctors who are dispensing medications (approximately 140 in 2007), resulting in an over-estimation compared with the data provided by other countries. Assistant pharmacists are also included in Iceland.

3.12.1 Pharmacists per 100 000 population, 2007 (or latest year available)

3.12.2 Change in the number of pharmacists per 100 000 population, 1990-2007 (or nearest year)

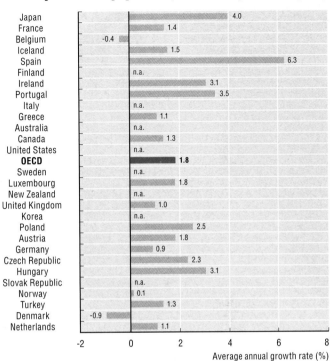

Country	3.12.1 (Per 100 000 population)	3.12.2 (Average annual growth rate %)
Japan	136	4.0
France	118	1.4
Belgium	116	-0.4
Iceland	114	1.5
Spain	108	6.3
Finland	105	n.a.
Ireland	104	3.1
Portugal	98	3.5
Italy	94	n.a.
Greece	88	1.1
Australia	87	n.a.
Canada	83	1.3
United States	80	n.a.
OECD	76	1.8
Sweden	73	n.a.
Luxembourg	72	1.8
New Zealand	68	n.a.
United Kingdom	68	1.0
Korea	65	n.a.
Poland	61	2.5
Austria	60	1.8
Germany	60	0.9
Czech Republic	56	2.3
Hungary	55	3.1
Slovak Republic	49	n.a.
Norway	46	0.1
Turkey	35	1.3
Denmark	21	-0.9
Netherlands	18	1.1

Per 100 000 population

Average annual growth rate (%)

Source: OECD Health Data 2009.

3.12.3 Pharmacies and other dispensaries of prescribed drugs per 100 000 population, selected OECD countries, 2007

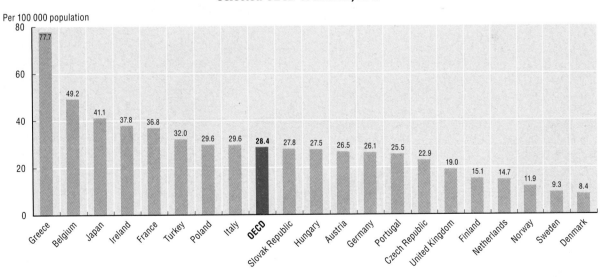

Per 100 000 population

Greece	77.7
Belgium	49.2
Japan	41.1
Ireland	37.8
France	36.8
Turkey	32.0
Poland	29.6
Italy	29.6
OECD	28.4
Slovak Republic	27.8
Hungary	27.5
Austria	26.5
Germany	26.1
Portugal	25.5
Czech Republic	22.9
United Kingdom	19.0
Finland	15.1
Netherlands	14.7
Norway	11.9
Sweden	9.3
Denmark	8.4

Source: Vogler et al. (2008) and Japanese Pharmaceutical Association (2008).

StatLink ⌐╗┗ http://dx.doi.org/10.1787/718350165545

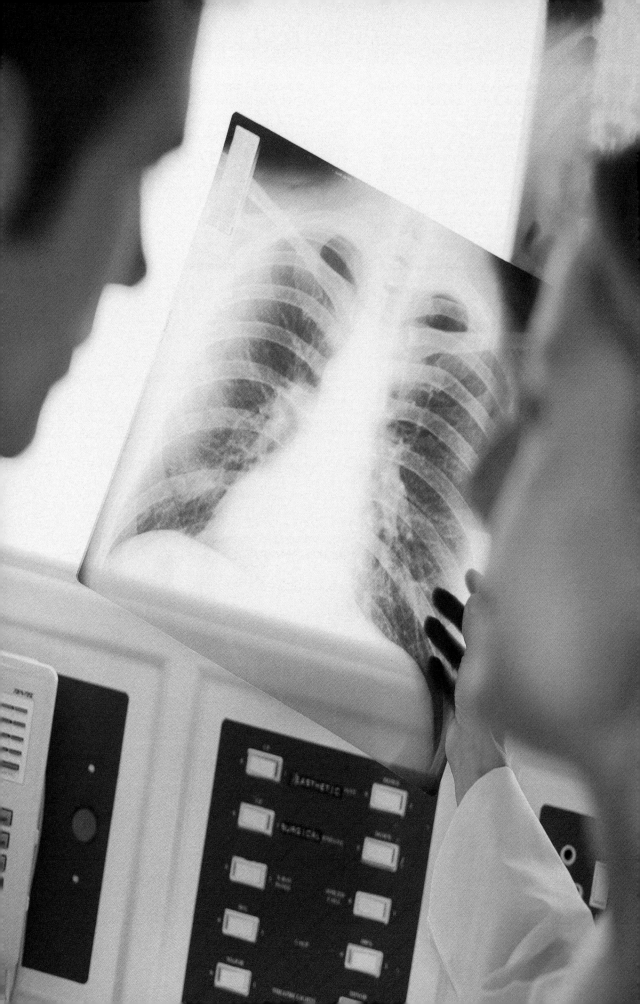

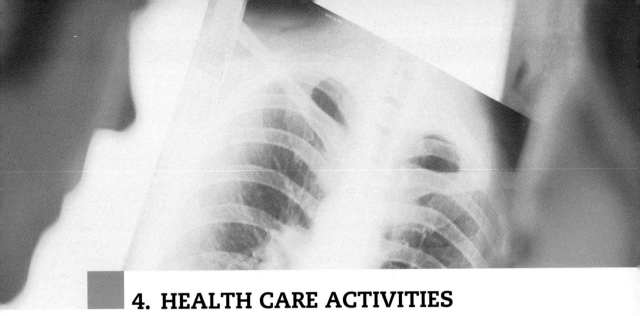

4. HEALTH CARE ACTIVITIES

Introduction

This chapter presents comparisons on the supply and use of different types of health services and goods in OECD countries. The provision of these services and the purchase of goods such as pharmaceuticals account for a large part of the health expenditure described in Chapter 7.

Indicators on a range of important health services are presented, including services provided in the primary care sector and in hospitals. The chapter begins by looking at levels and trends in the number of consultations with doctors, one of the most common services received by patients. The diffusion of modern medical technologies is generally considered to be one of the main drivers of rising health expenditure across OECD countries. The next section looks at the supply and use of two specific diagnostic technologies, medical resonance imaging (MRI) units and computed tomography (CT) scanners. The discussion then concentrates on hospital activities, a sector which continues to absorb the largest share of health spending in OECD countries, accounting for 35% to 40% of overall expenditure in many countries. The description of hospital services begins with a review of the availability of hospital beds, along with their rate of use. It then looks at the number of hospital discharges and the average length of stay in hospitals, for all conditions taken together as well as for a few selected conditions. Chapter 5 on "Quality of Care" compliments this by examining some of the reasons for hospitalisation that might be avoided, notably through better primary care for chronic conditions.

The next set of indicators in this chapter look more specifically at certain high-volume and high-cost procedures. These interventions include revascularisation procedures such as coronary artery bypass graft and coronary angioplasty for patients with ischemic heart diseases, dialysis and kidney transplants for patients suffering from end-stage renal failure, caesarean sections, and cataract surgeries. The main finding is that there are wide and unexplained variations in the use of different procedures across countries.

Over the past 20 years, research often originating from the United States as well as from other OECD countries has found that there can be an *overuse or inappropriate use* of certain medical or surgical interventions, in the sense that some interventions may be performed on patients for which scientific evidence suggests that the risks outweigh the expected benefits (OECD, 2004a). On the other hand, there can also be an *underuse* of certain services that are medically recommended for patients with certain conditions. Chapter 5 on "Quality of Care" provides several examples of the underuse of certain recommended services such as immunisation to prevent communicable diseases among children and other population groups. Chapter 6 on "Access to Care" adds information on *inequalities* in the use of certain health services among different socio-economic groups within countries.

In many countries, an important area of research has focussed on *regional* variations in medical and surgical procedure rates, which might provide some indication on the possible overuse or underuse of certain interventions in each country. In the United States, large variations have been reported across different States in the provision of common surgical procedures, such as knee replacement and cardiac surgeries, and these variations cannot be explained simply by differences in need (*Dartmouth Atlas of Health Care*, 2005). Geographical variations can also be found for non-surgical services, such as hospitalisations and physician visits. These findings indicate that there are also unexplained variations in clinical practices within each country, which are important to keep in mind in interpreting variations observed across countries.

The final section of this chapter looks at the volume of pharmaceutical consumption, focussing specifically on the use of drugs that treat diabetes and depression, drugs that lower cholesterol, and antibiotics. As is the case for health services, there may be an overuse or underuse of different pharmaceutical drugs for patients with various conditions. The aggregate data presented in this chapter does not allow any definitive conclusion on whether there is any inappropriate use of these pharmaceutical drugs, but they do show notable differences in prescribing levels across countries.

While this chapter covers many important health services, it does not cover long-term care services nor palliative care (end-of-life care). Information on consultations with dentists are included in Chapter 3 on the "Health Workforce", as part of the discussion on the number of dentists and how this might affect dentist consultations across countries. Information on certain public health services, such as immunisation rates and cancer screening rates, is provided in the next chapter on "Quality of Care", as they are deemed to be indicators of quality of care for communicable diseases and cancer.

4. HEALTH CARE ACTIVITIES

4.1. Consultations with doctors

Consultations with doctors can take place in doctors' offices or clinics, in hospital outpatient departments or, in some cases, in patients' own homes. In many European countries (*e.g.* Denmark, Italy, Netherlands, Norway, Portugal, Slovak Republic, Spain and United Kingdom), patients are required, or given incentives, to consult a general practitioner (GP) "gatekeeper" about any new episode of illness. The GP may then refer them to a specialist, if indicated. In other countries (*e.g.* Austria, Czech Republic, Iceland, Japan, Korea and Sweden), patients may approach specialists directly.

The number of doctor consultations per person per year ranges from over 11 in Japan and Korea, and in the Czech and Slovak Republics, to less than 3 in Mexico and Sweden (Figure 4.1.1). The OECD average is nearly 7 consultations per person per year. Cultural factors appear to play a role in explaining some of the variations across countries. For example, Japan and the Czech Republic are among the countries with the highest consultation rates although they report very different levels of health status and have very different physician density. But certain characteristics of health systems may also play a role in explaining these variations. There are signs that countries which pay their doctors mainly by fee-for-service tend to have above-average consultation rates (*e.g.* Japan and Korea), while countries which pay them mainly by salary tend to have below-average rates (*e.g.* Mexico and Sweden). However, there are examples of countries, such as Switzerland and the United States, where doctors are paid mainly by fee-for-service and where consultation rates are also below-average, suggesting that other factors also play a role. (See Table A.7 in Annex A for more information on the mode of payments of doctors in each country.)

In Sweden, the low number of doctor consultations may be explained partly by the fact that nurses play an important role in primary care, with many first contacts with patients carried out by nurses. Similarly, in Finland, nurses and other health professionals play an important role in providing primary care to patients in health centers, lowering the need for consultations with doctors (Bourgueil *et al.*, 2006).

The average number of doctor consultations has increased in most countries since 1990. The rise was particularly strong in Mexico, which started with a very low level in 1990. This can be at least partly explained by the rapid increase in physician density in Mexico during that period (see Indicator 3.2). In Sweden, the number of doctor consultations remained stable, while in Canada and the United Kingdom, it fell by about 1% per year between 1990 and 2007 (Figure 4.1.2). In Canada, the decrease can be attributed to the reduction in the proportion of consultations paid through fee-for-services, the only consultations identified and reported here.

Information on consultations can be used to estimate annual numbers of consultations per doctor in OECD countries. This estimate should not be taken as a measure of doctors' productivity, partly because consultations can vary in length and effectiveness and partly because it excludes the work doctors do on inpatients, administration and research. It is also subject to the comparability limitations reported in the box below on "Definition and deviations". Keeping these reservations in mind, this estimate varies nine-fold across OECD countries (Figure 4.1.3). Again, it is possible that some cultural factors play a part, because there is clustering of the two OECD Asian countries and the central and eastern European countries at the top of the ranking.

Chapter 6 on "Access to Care" provides additional information on disparities in the number of doctor consultations by income group (Indicator 6.5).

Definition and deviations

Consultations with doctors refer to the number of contacts with physicians (both generalists and specialists). There are variations across countries in the coverage of different types of consultations, notably the coverage of consultations in outpatient departments of hospitals.

The data come mainly from administrative sources, although in some countries (Italy, Netherlands, Spain, Switzerland, GP consultations in the United Kingdom and specialist consultations in New Zealand) the data come from health interview surveys. Estimates from administrative sources tend to be higher than those from surveys because of incorrect recall and non-response rates.

The figures for the Netherlands exclude contacts for maternal and child care. The data for Portugal and Turkey exclude visits to private practitioners, while those for the United Kingdom exclude private consultations with specialists.

4.1.1 Doctors consultations per capita, 2007 (or latest year available)

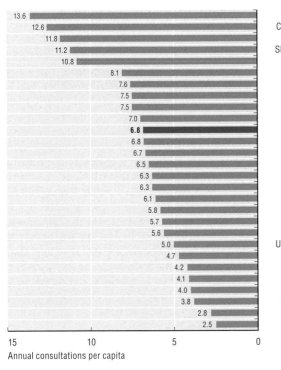

15   10   5   0
Annual consultations per capita

4.1.2 Change in the number of doctors consultations per capita, 1990-2007

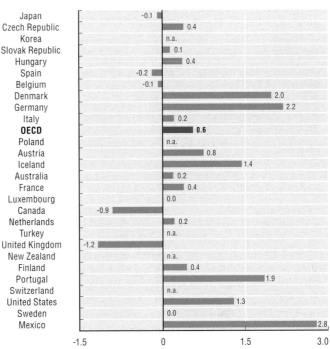

-1.5   0   1.5   3.0
Average annual growth rate (%)

4.1.3 Estimated number of consultations per doctor, 2007 (or latest year available)

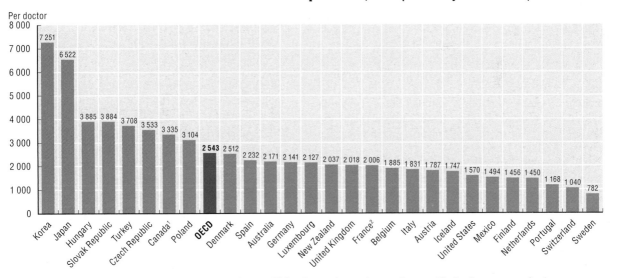

1. In Canada, the number of doctors only includes those paid fee-for-services to be consistent with the data on consultations.
2. In France, estimates of consultations in hospital out-patient departments have been added for more complete coverage.

Source: OECD Health Data 2009.

StatLink ⫘ http://dx.doi.org/10.1787/718370642522

4.2. Medical technologies (supply and use)

The diffusion of modern medical technologies is one main driver of rising health expenditure across OECD countries. This section presents data on the availability and intensity of use of two diagnostic technologies – computed tomography (CT) scanners and magnetic resonance imaging (MRI) units.

CT (or CAT, for computed axial tomography) scanners and MRI units help physicians diagnose a range of conditions by producing cross-sectional views of the inside of the body being scanned. Unlike conventional radiography and CT scanning, newer imaging technology used in MRI units do not expose patients to ionising radiation. The size and population density of a country is one of the factors affecting the number of equipment needed to respond to the demand.

The availability of CT scanners and MRI units has increased rapidly in most OECD countries over the past 15 years. Japan has, by far, the highest number of MRI and CT scanners per capita, followed by the United States for MRI units and by Australia for CT scanners (Figures 4.2.1 and 4.2.2). Some analysts attributed the rapid increase in MRI units in Japan, at least partly, to the lack of formal assessment of effectiveness or efficiency in purchasing decisions (Hisashige, 1992). At the other end of the scale, not surprisingly given their high cost, the number of MRI units and CT scanners were the lowest in Mexico and Hungary.

Data on the use of MRI and CT scanners are available for a smaller group of countries. Based on this more limited country coverage, the number of CT examinations ranges from highs of 228 scans per 1 000 population in the United States, followed by Luxembourg with 177 scans, to lows of 45 scans per 1 000 in France, although the figures in France and Australia do not include CT exams in public hospitals, thereby resulting in an under-estimation. The United States also has the highest number of MRI examinations per capita (Figures 4.2.3 and 4.2.4).

In the United States, some evidence suggests that there is a high risk of overuse of CT and MRI examinations. Between 1997 and 2006, the number of scans in the United States have increased dramatically while the occurrence of illnesses have remained constant (Smith-Bindman et al., 2008). Furthermore, to the extent that payment incentives allow doctors to benefit from exam referrals, this also increases the likelihood of overuse. Many studies have attempted to assess tangible medical benefits of the substantial increase in CT and MRI examinations in the United States but found no conclusive evidence suggesting such benefits (Baker et al., 2008).

Regarding the intensity of use of the equipment, as might be expected, there tends to be an inverse correlation between the availability of machines and the intensity of their use. In Hungary, Belgium and, to a lesser extent, the Czech Republic and Canada, fewer MRI units and CT scanners are associated with a more intensive use of each machine. Conversely, in the United States and Iceland, the high availability of MRI units and CT scanners is linked to less intensive use of each machine.

The inverted correlation between availability and intensity of use that is apparent in cross-country comparisons is less apparent when looking at trends in the number of new equipment installed and their utilisation rate in each country. In Canada, for instance, there has been an overall increase in both the availability and the intensity of use of MRI machines and CT scanners in recent years, indicating a substantial increase in the total number of exams. One explanation for the simultaneous increase in availability and intensity of use in Canada is that, in addition to a more intensive use of existing machines, the new machines serve regions that did not have access to the technology before (CIHI, 2008a).

Definition and deviations

MRI units and CT scanners relate to the number of equipment per million population. MRI exams and CT exams relate to the number of exams which can be divided either by the population or by the number of machines. Data are normally collected from both the hospital and the ambulatory sector.

However, data for some countries are under-estimated. Data on CT scanners and MRI units do not include those outside hospitals in some countries (Spain and Germany) or only a small number (France). For the United Kingdom, the data refer only to scanners in the public sector. For Australia, the number of MRI units (from 1999) includes only those eligible for reimbursement under Medicare, the universal public health system. In 1999, 60% of total MRI units were eligible for Medicare reimbursement. Also for Australia and France, data for CT and MRI exams refer only to utilization by out-patients and private in-patients (excluding those in public hospitals).

4.2.1 Number of MRI units per million population, 2007 (or latest year available)

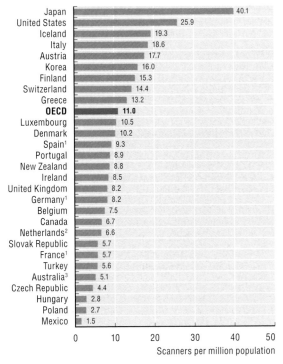

4.2.2 Number of CT scanners per million population, 2007 (or latest year available)

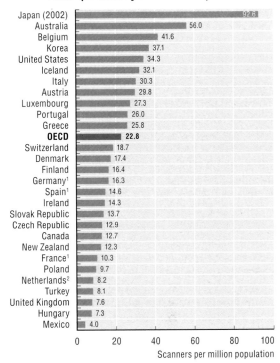

1. Only include equipment in hospitals (and a small number of equipment outside hospitals in France).   2. Only include the number of hospitals reporting to have at least one equipment.   3. Only MRI units eligible for reimbursement under Medicare.

4.2.3 Number of MRI exams per 1 000 population, 2007 (or latest year available)

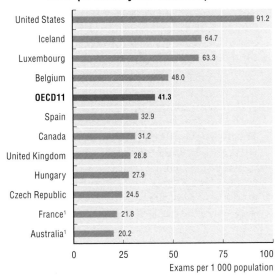

4.2.4 Number of CT exams per 1 000 population, 2007 (or latest year available)

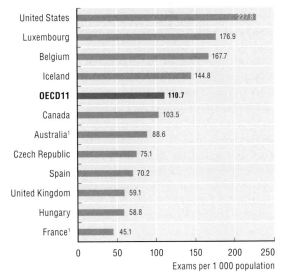

1. Only include exams for out-patients and private in-patients (excluding exams in public hospitals).

Source: OECD Health Data 2009.

StatLink 🔗🎏 *http://dx.doi.org/10.1787/718421073122*

4.3. Hospital beds (supply and use)

The number of hospital beds provides a measure of the resources available for delivering services to inpatients in hospitals. It does not capture, however, the capacity of hospitals to furnish same-day emergency or elective interventions. Furthermore, this section focuses solely on hospital beds allocated for acute care, not taking into accounts beds in psychiatric care or long-term care units.

The number of acute care hospital beds per capita is highest in Japan and Korea, with over seven beds per 1 000 population in 2007 (Figure 4.3.1). Both Japan and Korea have a problem of "social admission", that is, some "acute care" beds may be devoted to long-term care use (Hurst, 2007). The number of acute care beds is also well above the OECD average in Austria and Germany. It is the lowest in Mexico, followed by Sweden and Spain.

The number of acute care beds in hospitals has decreased in most OECD countries. On average across countries, the number fell from 4.7 per 1 000 population in 1995 to 3.8 in 2007. Only in Korea and Turkey has the number of acute care beds grown between 1995 and 2007. In Korea, the marked increase can be explained by the use of acute care beds for long-term care, the lack of capacity planning for hospital beds, and investment incentives in the private for-profit hospital system (OECD, 2003b).

The reduction in the number of acute care hospital beds observed in most countries has been driven, at least partly, by progress in medical technology which has enabled a move to day surgery and a reduced need for hospitalisation. In addition, cost-containment policies have often targeted the hospital sector, which remains the largest health spending category in nearly all OECD countries (see Indicator 7.3 "Health expenditure by function"). The reduction in the availability of hospital beds has been accompanied in many countries by a reduction in hospital admissions and the average length of stay (see Indicator 4.5 "Average length of stay in hospitals").

In several countries, the reduction in the number of acute care hospital beds has also been accompanied by an increase in their occupancy rates. The occupancy rate of acute care beds stood at 75% on average across OECD countries in 2007, slightly above the 1995 level (Figure 4.3.2). Canada, Norway, Ireland, Switzerland, and the United Kingdom had the highest occupancy

rates in 2007. All of these countries have fewer acute care beds than most other OECD countries. On the other hand, Mexico and the Netherlands have the lowest occupancy rates, with a rate below 65% in 2007. In the Netherlands, the occupancy rate has decreased sharply since 1995 while the number of acute care beds also fell.

Definition and deviations

Acute care hospital beds normally only include beds available for "curative care" as defined in the OECD Manual *A System of Health Accounts* (OECD, 2000). However, the functions of care included/excluded in "acute care" vary across countries and across time – for example the extent to which beds allocated for long-term care, rehabilitation and palliative care are excluded – thereby limiting data comparability. Several countries (*e.g.* Australia, Austria, Canada, Germany, Ireland, Luxembourg, Netherlands, Poland, Portugal, Spain, Switzerland, Turkey and the United States) report as acute beds all beds located in "general" or "acute care" hospitals. Also, some acute beds may be used for purposes such as long-term care (*e.g.* in Japan and Korea). In the Netherlands, the calculation of occupancy rates is based on the number of licensed beds rather than the number of available beds, resulting in a slight under-estimation (the number of licensed beds can be 2 to 10% higher than the number of available beds). Private sector beds are not included, or only partially included, in Hungary and Ireland. Data for Finland are not based on an actual count of beds, but rather estimated by dividing the number of hospital days for acute care by the total number of days in the year (365); this leads to an under-estimation, given that occupancy rate is lower than the assumed 100% rate.

The occupancy rate for acute care beds is calculated as the number of hospital bed-days related to acute care divided by the number of available acute care beds (which is multiplied by the number of days, 365).

4.3.1 Acute care hospital beds per 1 000 population, 1995 and 2007 (or nearest year available)

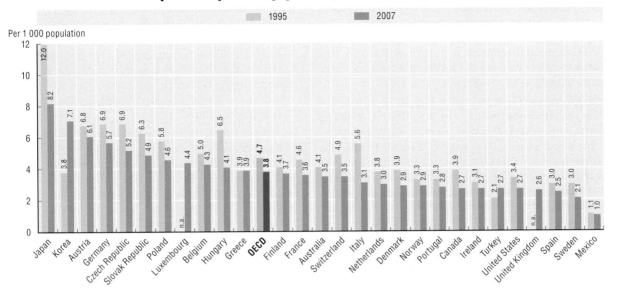

4.3.2 Occupancy rate of acute care hospital beds, 1995 and 2007 (or nearest year available)

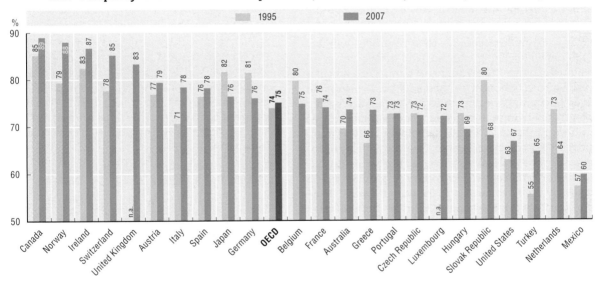

Source: OECD Health Data 2009.

StatLink 🔊 http://dx.doi.org/10.1787/718421246808

Hospital discharge rates are a measure of the number of people who need to stay overnight in a hospital each year. Together with the average length of stay, they are important measures of hospital activities. However, overall discharge rates do not take into account differences in case-mix (the mix of the conditions leading to hospitalisation).

Hospital discharge rates are the highest in Austria and France, although the high rate in France is partly explained by the inclusion of some same-day separations (Figure 4.4.1). Discharge rates are also high in Germany, the Czech Republic, Poland and the Slovak Republic. They are the lowest in Mexico and Canada. In general, those countries that have more hospital beds tend to have higher discharge rates and *vice versa* (see Indicator 4.3 "Hospital beds").

Over the past decade, discharge rates have increased in some countries, most notably in Korea and Turkey which started with relatively low levels. They remained stable in other countries such as Australia, Spain and the United States, while they fell significantly in Canada, Italy and Iceland. In Canada, a marked decline in the number of hospitalisations was accompanied by a strong rise in the number of day surgeries in or outside hospitals (CIHI, 2007).

Elderly populations account for a disproportionately high percentage of overall hospital discharges in all countries. In the United States, 24% of all hospital discharges in 2006 concerned people aged 75 years and over, up from 16% in 1990. However, population ageing may be a less important factor in explaining changes in hospitalisation rates than evolving clinical practices linked to advances in medical technologies. For example, hospital stays involving at least one revascularisation procedure (a coronary angioplasty or a coronary artery bypass graft) for people aged 75 to 84 doubled between 1990 and 2006 in the United States (NCHS, 2009).

On average across OECD countries, the main conditions leading to hospitalisation in 2007 were circulatory diseases which include ischemic heart disease, stroke and other diseases (13% of all discharges), pregnancy and childbirth (11%), diseases of the digestive system (10%), injuries and other external causes (9%), and cancers (9%).

Austria has the highest discharge rate for circulatory diseases, followed by Germany, Hungary and Poland (Figure 4.4.2). The high rate in Hungary is associated with high mortality rate from circulatory diseases which may be used as a proxy indicator for the occurrence of these diseases (see Indicator 1.4 "Mortality from heart disease and stroke"). This is less the case for the other three countries that have high discharge rates. In Germany, the high discharge rate for ischemic heart disease is associated with the highest rate of revascularisation procedures (see Indicator 4.6 "Cardiac procedures").

Austria, Hungary, Germany and Poland also have the highest discharge rates for cancer (Figure 4.4.3). The high rate in Hungary and Poland is associated with high mortality rates from cancer, which may also be used as a proxy for the occurrence of the disease (see Indicator 1.5 "Mortality from cancer"). However, this is not the case for Austria and Germany. In Austria, the high rate is associated with a high rate of hospital readmissions for further investigation and treatment of cancer patients (European Commission, 2008a).

Definition and deviations

Discharge is defined as the release of a patient who has stayed at least one night in hospital. It includes deaths in hospital following inpatient care. Same-day separations are usually excluded, with the exceptions of Canada, France and the United States which include some same-day separations.

Healthy babies born in hospitals are excluded completely (or almost completely) from hospital discharge rates in several countries (*e.g.* Australia, Canada, Finland, Greece, Ireland, Japan, Korea, Luxembourg, Mexico, Norway, Sweden, Turkey). Ireland also excludes discharges related to pregnancy and childbirth and certain conditions originating in the perinatal period.

Some countries do not cover all hospitals. For instance, data for Denmark, Ireland, Mexico, Poland and the United Kingdom are restricted to public or publicly-funded hospitals only. Data for Portugal relate only to hospitals on the mainland (excluding the Islands of Azores and Madeira).

4.4.1 Hospital discharges per 1 000 population, 2007 (or latest year available)

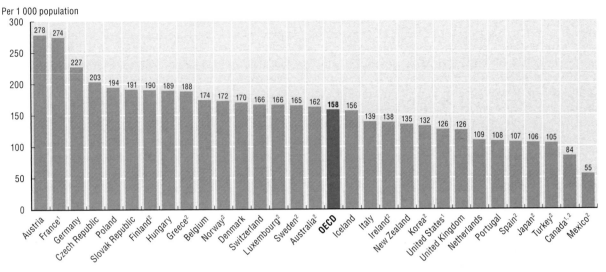

1. Includes same-day separations.
2. Excludes discharges of healthy babies born in hospital.

4.4.2 Hospital discharges for circulatory diseases per 1 000 population, 2007 (or latest year available)

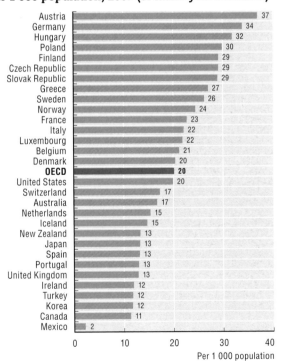

4.4.3 Hospital discharges for cancers per 1 000 population, 2007 (or latest year available)

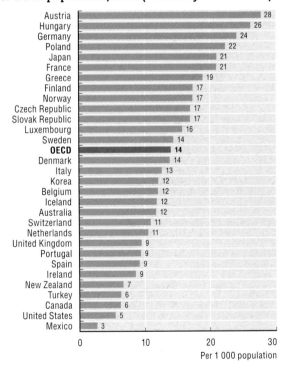

Source: OECD Health Data 2009.

StatLink ᐧᐧᒪ http://dx.doi.org/10.1787/718432575088

4.5. Average length of stay in hospitals

The average length of stay in hospitals (ALOS) is often treated as an indicator of efficiency. All other things being equal, a shorter stay will reduce the cost per discharge and shift care from inpatient to less expensive post-acute settings. However, shorter stays tend to be more service intensive and more costly per day. Too short a length of stay could also cause adverse effect on health outcomes, or reduce the comfort and recovery of the patient. If this leads to a rising readmission rate, costs per episode of illness may fall little, or even rise.

In 2007, the average length of stay for acute care for all conditions combined was the lowest in some Nordic countries (Denmark, Finland, Sweden), Mexico and Turkey (less than five days), and the highest in Japan (19 days), followed by Germany and Switzerland (almost eight days). The OECD average was 6.5 days (Figure 4.5.1). Several factors can explain these cross-country differences. Short stays in Finland are linked, at least partly, to the availability of beds for convalescent patients in health centres (OECD, 2005b). Conversely, the abundant supply of beds and the structure of hospital payments in Japan may provide hospitals with incentives to keep patients longer (see Indicator 4.3 "Hospital beds"). Financial incentives inherent in hospital payment methods can also influence length of stay in other countries. For example, predominant bed-day payments in Switzerland have encouraged long stays in hospitals (OECD and WHO, 2006).

The average length of stay for acute care has fallen in nearly all OECD countries – from 8.7 days in 1995 to 6.5 days in 2007 on average across OECD countries (Figure 4.5.1). It fell particularly quickly in those countries that had relatively high levels in 1995 (Japan, Germany, Netherlands, Switzerland, Czech Republic, Slovak Republic, Hungary and Poland). Several factors explain this decline, including the use of less invasive surgical procedures, changes in hospital payment methods to prospective pricing systems, and the expansion of early discharge programmes which enable patients to return to their home to receive follow-up care.

Focusing on average length of stay for specific diseases or conditions can remove some of the heterogeneity arising from different mix and severity of acute care conditions across countries. Figure 4.5.3 shows that ALOS following a normal delivery ranges from less than two days in Mexico, Turkey, the United Kingdom and Canada, to five days or more in the Slovak Republic, Hungary, Switzerland and the Czech Republic. ALOS for normal delivery has become shorter in nearly all countries over the past decade, dropping from 4.3 days in 1995 to 3.2 days in 2007 on average across OECD countries.

Lengths of stay following acute myocardial infarction (AMI, or heart attack) also declined over the past decade. In 2007, ALOS following AMI was the lowest in Turkey, some of the Nordic countries (Norway, Sweden and Denmark) and the United States (less than six days). It was 11 days or more in Finland and Germany (Figure 4.5.2). Care is however required in making cross-country comparisons. For example, ALOS in Finland may include patients originally admitted for AMI but who are no longer receiving acute care, and might therefore be considered long-term care patients (Moïse et al., 2003).

Definition and deviations

Average length of stay (ALOS) for acute care refers to the average number of days that patients spend in hospital. It is generally measured by dividing the total number of days stayed by all patients in acute-care units in hospital during a year by the number of admissions or discharges.

The definition of "acute care" includes all the functions of care covered under "curative care" as defined in the OECD Manual, A System of Health Accounts (OECD, 2000). However, there are variations across countries in the functions of care included/excluded in "acute care", thereby limiting data comparability (e.g. whether or not beds for rehabilitation, palliative care and long-term care are included).

In the calculation of ALOS, days and discharges of healthy babies born in hospitals are excluded or only partially counted in some countries. Including healthy newborns would reduce the ALOS in these countries (e.g. by about half-a-day in Canada).

4.5.1 Average length of stay for acute care, 1995 and 2007 (or nearest year)

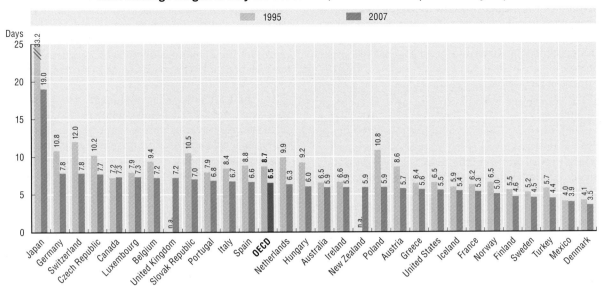

Legend: 1995, 2007

4.5.2 Average length of stay following acute myocardial infarction (AMI), 2007 (or latest year available)

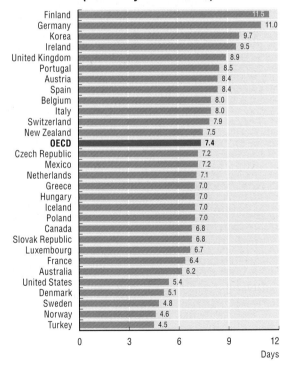

Country	Days
Finland	11.5
Germany	11.0
Korea	9.7
Ireland	9.5
United Kingdom	8.9
Portugal	8.5
Austria	8.4
Spain	8.4
Belgium	8.0
Italy	8.0
Switzerland	7.9
New Zealand	7.5
OECD	7.4
Czech Republic	7.2
Mexico	7.2
Netherlands	7.1
Greece	7.0
Hungary	7.0
Iceland	7.0
Poland	7.0
Canada	6.8
Slovak Republic	6.8
Luxembourg	6.7
France	6.4
Australia	6.2
United States	5.4
Denmark	5.1
Sweden	4.8
Norway	4.6
Turkey	4.5

4.5.3 Average length of stay for normal delivery, 2007 (or latest year available)

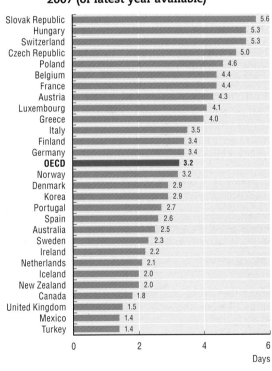

Country	Days
Slovak Republic	5.6
Hungary	5.3
Switzerland	5.3
Czech Republic	5.0
Poland	4.6
Belgium	4.4
France	4.4
Austria	4.3
Luxembourg	4.1
Greece	4.0
Italy	3.5
Finland	3.4
Germany	3.4
OECD	3.2
Norway	3.2
Denmark	2.9
Korea	2.9
Portugal	2.7
Spain	2.6
Australia	2.5
Sweden	2.3
Ireland	2.2
Netherlands	2.1
Iceland	2.0
New Zealand	2.0
Canada	1.8
United Kingdom	1.5
Mexico	1.4
Turkey	1.4

Source: OECD Health Data 2009.

StatLink ᴍˢᴸ http://dx.doi.org/10.1787/718461788142

4. HEALTH CARE ACTIVITIES

4.6. Cardiac procedures (coronary bypass and angioplasty)

Heart diseases are a leading cause of hospitalisation and death in OECD countries (see Indicator 1.4). Coronary artery bypass graft and angioplasty are two revascularisation procedures that have revolutionised the treatment of ischemic heart diseases in recent decades.

There is considerable variation across countries in the use of coronary bypass surgery and angioplasty (Figure 4.6.1). Germany, the United States and Belgium have the highest rates of angioplasty in 2007. These three countries also have the highest rates of coronary artery bypass grafts. While at the individual patient level, coronary angioplasty may be a substitute for coronary bypass surgery, at the aggregate level, a higher rate of angioplasty in one country is *not* associated with a lower rate of bypass surgery. Countries that perform high rates of one type of revascularisation procedure also tend to perform high rates of the other.

In Belgium, the high rate of both coronary angioplasty and bypass surgery can be partly attributed to a sizeable number of non-residents receiving these treatments in Belgian hospitals. In 2006, 2.5% of people who received an angioplasty on an inpatient basis in Belgium were non-residents; this proportion reached about 4% for people receiving a bypass surgery (European Commission, 2008a).

The use of angioplasty has increased rapidly since 1990 in most OECD countries, overtaking bypass surgery as the preferred method of revascularisation around the mid-1990s – about the same time that the first published trials of the efficacy of coronary stenting began to appear (Moïse, 2003). The trend rise has also been supported by the introduction of drug-eluting stents and the decreased use of coronary bypass in most OECD countries. In most countries, angioplasty now accounts for between 65% and 80% of total revascularisations (Figure 4.6.2). Although angioplasty has replaced in many cases bypass surgery, it is not a perfect substitute since bypass surgery is still the preferred method for treating patients with multiple-vessel obstructions, diabetes and other conditions (Taggart, 2009).

A number of reasons can explain cross-country variations in the number of revascularisation procedures, including: i) differences in the incidence and prevalence of ischemic heart diseases; ii) differences in the capacity to deliver and pay for these procedures; iii) differences in clinical treatment guidelines and practices; and iv) coding and reporting practices.

The large variations in the number of revascularisation procedures across countries do not seem to be closely related to the incidence of ischemic heart disease (IHD), as measured by IHD mortality (Figure 4.6.3). IHD mortality in Germany is only slightly higher than the average across OECD countries, but Germany has the highest rate of revascularisation procedures. On the other hand, IHD mortality in Hungary and Finland is well above the OECD average, while revascularisation rates are below average. Some countries may be under-utilising revascularisation procedures, while others may be carrying out too many costly interventions which have little benefit.

Definition and deviations

A coronary bypass is the grafting of veins and/or arteries to bypass an obstructed coronary artery. It may involve bypassing only one coronary artery, but multiple coronary artery bypasses are more common. Coronary angioplasty involves the threading of a catheter with a balloon attached to the tip through the arterial system, usually started in the femoral artery in the leg, into the diseased coronary artery. The balloon is inflated to distend the coronary artery at the point of obstruction. The placement of a stent to keep the artery open accompanies the majority of angioplasties. Drug-eluting stents (a stent that gradually releases drugs) are increasingly being used to stem the growth of scar-like tissue surrounding the stent.

The data relate to inpatient procedures, normally counting *all* procedures. However, classification systems and registration practices vary across countries, and the same procedure can be recorded differently (*e.g.* an angioplasty with the placement of a stent can be counted as one or two procedures). Some countries report only the *main* procedure (or the number of *patients* receiving one or more procedures), resulting in an under-estimation of the total number. This is the case for the Netherlands, Spain and the United States (for coronary bypass). In Ireland, the data only include activities in publicly-funded hospitals (it is estimated that over 10% of all hospital activity in Ireland is undertaken in private hospitals). For all countries, the data do not include coronary angioplasties performed on an ambulatory basis.

4.6.1 Coronary revascularisation procedures, per 100 000 population, 2007 (or latest year available)

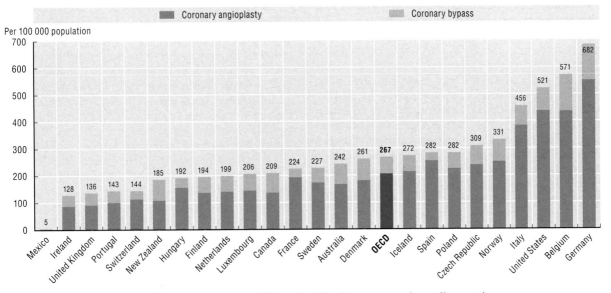

Legend: ▰ Coronary angioplasty ▱ Coronary bypass

Per 100 000 population

Values (left to right): Mexico 5, Ireland 128, United Kingdom 136, Portugal 143, Switzerland 144, New Zealand 185, Hungary 192, Finland 194, Netherlands 199, Luxembourg 206, Canada 209, France 224, Sweden 227, Australia 242, Denmark 261, **OECD 267**, Iceland 272, Spain 282, Poland 282, Czech Republic 309, Norway 331, Italy 456, United States 521, Belgium 571, Germany 682

Note: Some of the variations across countries are due to different classification systems and recording practices.

4.6.2 Coronary angioplasty as a percentage of total revascularisation procedures, 1990-2007

Legend: —— Australia – – – France –·–·– Italy ······ United States **—— OECD12**

% of total revascularisation procedures

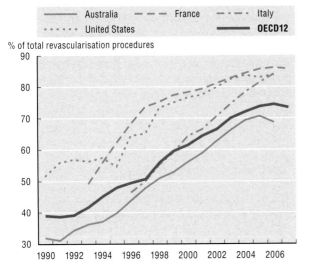

4.6.3 Ischemic heart disease mortality and coronary revascularisation procedures, 2006

IHD, age-standardised death rates, per 100 000 population

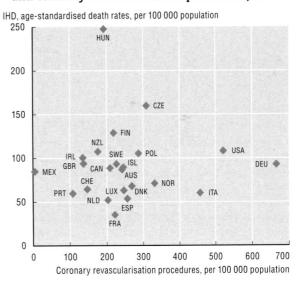

Coronary revascularisation procedures, per 100 000 population

Source: OECD Health Data 2009.

StatLink ⬛⬛ *http://dx.doi.org/10.1787/718488133776*

End-stage renal failure (ESRF) is a condition in which the kidneys are permanently impaired and can no longer function normally. Some of the main risk factors for end-stage renal failure include diabetes and hypertension, two conditions which are generally becoming more prevalent in OECD countries. In the United States, diabetes and hypertension alone accounted for over 60% of the primary diagnoses for all ESRF patients (37% for diabetes and 24% for hypertension) (USRDS, 2008). When patients reach end-stage renal failure, they require treatment either in the form of dialysis or through kidney transplants. Treatment in the form of dialysis tends to be more costly and results in a poorer quality of life for patients than a successful kidney transplant, because of the recurrent nature of dialysis.

Taking into account both types of treatment, the proportion of people treated for end-stage renal failure has increased at a rate of almost 6% per year on average across OECD countries over the past two decades (Figure 4.7.2). This translates into a more than three-fold increase in the prevalence of treatment for ESRF in 2007 compared with 1985. In 2007, Japan and the United States reported the highest rates, with more than 160 ESRF patients per 100 000 population (Figure 4.7.1). They were followed by Portugal which registered the highest growth rate since 1985. It is not clear why these countries report such strong rates of treatment for ESRF, but it does not seem to be solely or mainly related to a higher prevalence of diabetes, which is not particularly higher in these countries compared with other OECD countries (see Indicator 1.12 "Diabetes prevalence and incidence").

In most OECD countries, a majority of ESRF patients are being treated through dialysis as opposed to receiving a kidney transplant. This can be attributed to the fact that while the prevalence of people suffering from end-stage renal failure has strongly increased in many countries, the number of transplants has remained limited by the number of donors. The exceptions are Finland, Iceland and the Netherlands which have a relatively low level of ESRF patients overall.

The proportion of people undergoing dialysis is much higher in Japan and, to a lesser extent, in the United States, than in other countries (Figure 4.7.3). In Japan, this is partly related to very low rates of kidney transplants, meaning that nearly all Japanese ESRF patients are treated through dialysis. In all countries, there has been a large rise in the number of persons undergoing dialysis over the past 20 years.

Given the supply constraints, kidney transplants are normally performed on patients with end-stage renal failure when these persons cannot live without long and hard dialysis sessions. When successful, these transplants allow people to live again almost normally, without strict diet and activity limitation. Advances in surgical techniques and the development of new drugs preventing rejection have made it possible to carry out more transplants, and to improve their rate of success, than was the case 20 years ago. The prevalence of people living with a functioning kidney transplant has regularly increased since 1985 in all countries with available data. The OECD average rose from eight to 34 people with a functioning kidney transplant per 100 000 population between 1985 and 2007 (Figure 4.7.4). In 2007, the United States, Portugal and Austria reported the highest rates, with more than 45 people with a functioning kidney transplant per 100 000 population. On the other hand, the proportion of people having received a kidney transplant was the lowest in Japan, followed by Korea and the Slovak Republic.

In many countries, waiting lists to receive a kidney transplant have increased, as the demand for transplants has outpaced greatly the number of donors. The rate of transplants is also affected by cultural factors and traditions; transplants may still be less accepted in certain countries such as Japan.

Definition and deviations

The number of patients treated for end-stage renal failure refers to the number of patients at the end of the year who are receiving different forms of renal replacement therapy: haemodialysis/haemoinfiltration, intermittent peritoneal dialysis, continuous ambulatory peritoneal dialysis, continuous cyclical peritoneal dialysis, or living with a functioning kidney transplant.

4.7.1 Patients treated for end-stage renal failure, by type of treatment, 2007 (or latest year available)

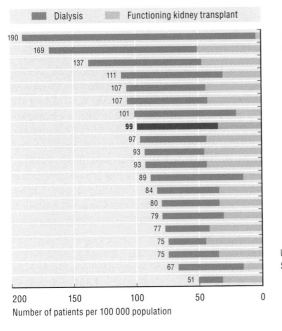

4.7.2 Rise in the prevalence of people treated for end-stage renal failure, 1985-2007

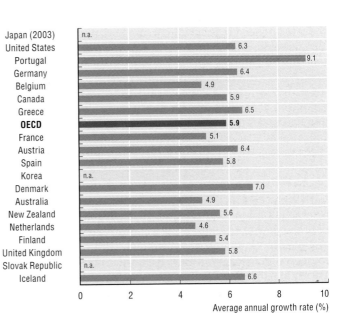

4.7.3 Prevalence of patients undergoing dialysis, 1985 and 2007 (or nearest year)

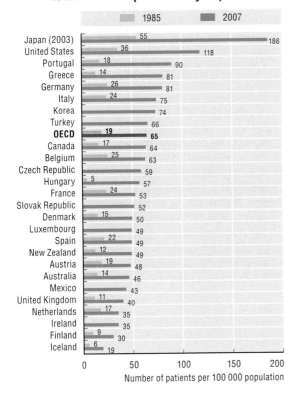

4.7.4 Prevalence of patients living with a functioning kidney transplant, 1985 and 2007 (or nearest year)

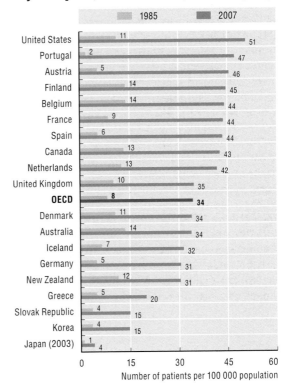

Source: OECD Health Data 2009.

StatLink http://dx.doi.org/10.1787/718535684543

Rates of caesarean delivery (as a percentage of all live births) have increased in all OECD countries in recent decades. Reasons for the increase include reductions in the risk of caesarean delivery, malpractice liability concerns, scheduling convenience for both physicians and patients, and changes in the physician-patient relationship, among others. Nonetheless, caesarean delivery continues to result in increased maternal mortality, maternal and infant morbidity, and increased complications for subsequent deliveries (Minkoff and Chervenak, 2003; Bewley and Cockburn, 2002; Villar *et al.*, 2006). These concerns, combined with the greater financial cost, raise the question of whether the costs of caesarean delivery may exceed the benefits.

In 2007, the caesarean section rate varied significantly across OECD countries (Figure 4.8.1), ranging from lows of 14% in the Netherlands to highs of nearly 40% in Italy and Mexico. The rates were also high (30% or more) in Australia, Hungary, Korea, Portugal, Switzerland, Turkey and the United States. The average across OECD countries was 26%. In the Netherlands, where home births are a usual option for women with low-risk pregnancies, 30% of all births occurred at home in 2004 (Euro-Peristat, 2008).

The increase in caesarean section rates slowed or even reversed in some OECD countries during the 1990s, as a result of changes in obstetrical practice including trial of labor (*i.e.* when a woman attempts labor and normal delivery after having a caesarean) to reduce the number of repeat caesareans (Lagrew and Adashek, 1998). But caesarean rates soon resumed their upward trend, due in part to reports of complications from trial of labor and continued changes in patient preferences (Sachs *et al.*, 1999). Other trends, such as increases in first births among older women and the rise in multiple births resulting from assisted reproduction, also contributed to the global rise in caesarean deliveries.

The increase in caesarean rates since 1997 has been rapid in most OECD countries (Figures 4.8.2 and 4.8.3). Average annual growth rates of 4% or more were recorded in 12 OECD countries, with the highest growth rates in Austria, the Slovak Republic, Luxembourg, Denmark, Ireland and the Czech Republic. Caesarean section rates have grown at an annual rate of 3.9% across OECD countries from 1997 to 2007. Finland and

Iceland have had the lowest growth rates and are among the countries with the lowest caesarean rates in 2007.

The continued rise in caesarean deliveries is only partly related to changes in medical indications. A study of caesarean delivery trends in the United States found that the proportion of "no indicated risk" caesareans rose from 3.7% of all births in 1996 to 5.5% in 2001 (Declercq *et al.*, 2005). In France, a 2008 study by the French Hospital Federation found higher caesarean rates in private for-profit facilities than in public facilities, even though the latter are designed to deal with more complicated pregnancies (FHF, 2008). A review of caesarean delivery practice in Latin American countries in the late 1990s similarly found higher caesarean rates in private hospitals than in public or social security hospitals (Belizan *et al.*, 1999).

While caesarean delivery is clearly required in some circumstances, the benefits of caesarean *versus* vaginal delivery for normal uncomplicated deliveries continue to be debated. Professional associations of obstetricians and gynaecologists in countries such as Canada now encourage the promotion of normal childbirth without interventions such as caesarean sections (Society of Obstetricians and Gynaecologists of Canada *et al.*, 2008).

Definition and deviations

Caesarean section rate is the number of caesareans per 100 live births.

In Portugal, the denominator is only the number of live births which took place in National Health Service Hospitals on the mainland (resulting in an over-estimation of caesarean rates). In Mexico, the number of caesarean sections is estimated based on public hospital reports and data obtained from National Health Surveys. Estimation is required to correct for under-reporting of caesarean deliveries in private facilities. The combined number of caesarean deliveries is then divided by the total number of live births as estimated by the National Population Council.

4.8.1 Caesarean sections per 100 live births, 2007 (or latest year available)

4.8.2 Rise in caesarean sections per 100 live births, 1997-2007 (or nearest year)

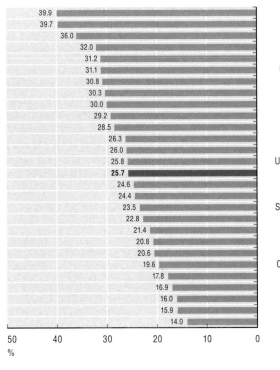

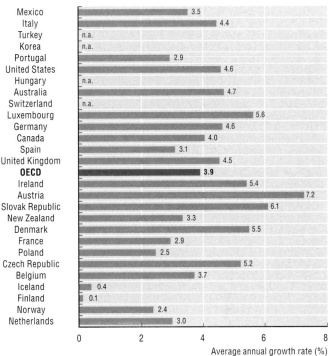

	4.8.1 (%)	4.8.2 (Average annual growth rate %)
Mexico	39.9	3.5
Italy	39.7	4.4
Turkey	36.0	n.a.
Korea	32.0	n.a.
Portugal	31.2	2.9
United States	31.1	4.6
Hungary	30.8	n.a.
Australia	30.3	4.7
Switzerland	30.0	n.a.
Luxembourg	29.2	5.6
Germany	28.5	4.6
Canada	26.3	4.0
Spain	26.0	3.1
United Kingdom	25.8	4.5
OECD	**25.7**	**3.9**
Ireland	24.6	5.4
Austria	24.4	7.2
Slovak Republic	23.5	6.1
New Zealand	22.8	3.3
Denmark	21.4	5.5
France	20.8	2.9
Poland	20.6	2.5
Czech Republic	19.6	5.2
Belgium	17.8	3.7
Iceland	16.9	0.4
Finland	16.0	0.1
Norway	15.9	2.4
Netherlands	14.0	3.0

4.8.3 Caesarean sections per 100 live births, 1990-2007 (or nearest year)

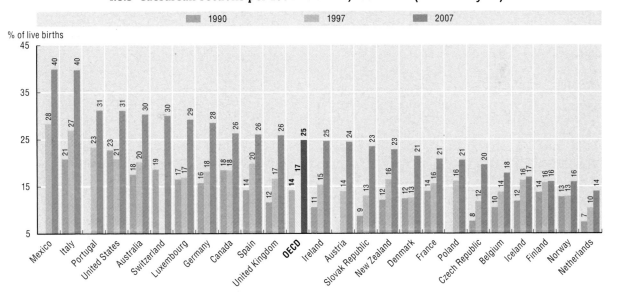

Legend: 1990, 1997, 2007

% of live births

	1990	1997	2007
Mexico	28		40
Italy	21	27	40
Portugal	23	23	31
United States	21		31
Australia	18	20	30
Switzerland	19		30
Luxembourg	17	17	29
Germany	16	18	28
Canada	18	18	26
Spain	14	20	26
United Kingdom	12	17	26
OECD	**14**	**17**	**25**
Ireland	11	15	25
Austria	14		24
Slovak Republic	9	13	23
New Zealand	12	16	23
Denmark	12	13	21
France	14	16	21
Poland	16		21
Czech Republic	8	12	20
Belgium	10	14	18
Iceland	12	16	17
Finland	14	16	16
Norway	13	13	16
Netherlands	7	10	14

Source: OECD Health Data 2009.

StatLink ᴍˢᴸ *http://dx.doi.org/10.1787/718547335063*

4. HEALTH CARE ACTIVITIES

4.9. Cataract surgeries

In the past 20 years, the number of surgical procedures carried out on a day care basis has steadily grown in OECD countries. Advances in medical technologies, particularly the diffusion of less invasive surgical interventions, and better anaesthetics have made this development possible. These innovations have improved effectiveness and patient safety. They also help to reduce the unit cost of interventions by shortening the length of stay. However, the overall impact on cost depends on the extent to which any greater use of these procedures may be offset by a reduction in unit cost, taking into account the cost of post-acute care and community health services.

Cataract surgery provides a good example of a high volume surgery which is now carried out predominantly on a day care basis in most OECD countries. It has now become the most frequent surgical procedure in many OECD countries.

The number of cataract procedures per capita ranges from a low of 59 per 100 000 population in Mexico to a high of 1 722 per 100 000 population in Belgium (Figure 4.9.1). Both demand factors (including an older population structure) and supply factors (such as the capacity to perform the intervention in hospital and outside hospital) provide explanations for these cross-country variations. However, the comparability of data is also limited by registration problems, particularly the lack of registration of day surgeries carried outside hospitals in some countries, which explain the low rates in Ireland and Poland. The very high rate in countries such as Belgium may be explained partly by the registration of more than one procedure per surgery.

The volume of cataract surgeries has grown over the past decade in most OECD countries. Population ageing is one of the factors behind this trend rise, but the proven success, safety and cost-effectiveness of cataract surgery as a day care procedure has probably been a more important factor (Fedorowicz *et al.*, 2004).

Cataract surgeries are now predominantly performed on a day care basis in most OECD countries. Day surgery accounts for 90% or more of all cataract surgeries in a majority of countries for which data are available (Figure 4.9.2). However, the diffusion of day surgery is still relatively low in some countries, such as Poland and Hungary. This may be explained by more advantageous reimbursement for in-patient stays, national regulations, and obstacles to changing individual practices of surgeons and anaesthetists (Castoro *et al.*, 2007), together with limitations in data coverage. In

France, the share of cataract surgeries carried out on a same-day basis has increased rapidly over the past decade, from 19% in 1997 to 63% in 2007, but it still remains below that of many other OECD countries. In several OECD countries, there may still be room to increase the share of operations carried out on a same-day basis.

In Sweden, there is evidence that cataract surgeries are now being performed on patients suffering from less severe vision problems compared to five or ten years ago. This raises the question of how the needs of these patients should be prioritised relative to other patient populations (Swedish Association of Local Authorities and Regions and National Board of Health and Welfare, 2008).

Definition and deviations

Cataract surgeries consist of removing the lens of the eye (because of the presence of cataracts which are partially or completely clouding the lens) and replacing it with an artificial lens. The surgery may be carried out as day cases or as in-patient cases (involving an overnight stay in hospital). Same-day interventions may either be performed in a hospital or in a clinic. However, the data for most countries only include interventions carried out in hospitals. Caution is therefore required in making cross-country comparisons of available data, given the incomplete coverage of day surgeries in several countries.

Denmark only includes cataract surgeries carried out in public hospitals, excluding procedures carried out in the ambulatory sector and in private hospitals. In Ireland too, the data cover only procedures in public hospitals (it is estimated that over 10% of all hospital activity in Ireland is undertaken in private hospitals). The data for Spain only partially include the activities in private hospitals.

Classification systems and registration practices for cataract surgeries also vary across countries, for instance whether they are counted as one intervention involving at least two steps (removal or the lens and replacement with an artificial lens) or as two separate interventions.

4.9.1 Number of cataract surgeries, inpatient and day cases, per 100 000 population, 1997 and 2007 (or nearest year)

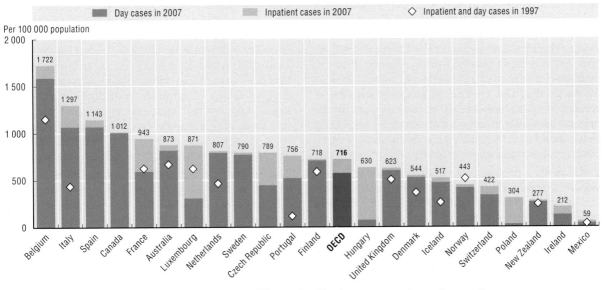

Note: Some of the variations across countries are due to different classification systems and recording practices.

4.9.2 Share of cataract surgeries carried out as day cases, 1997 and 2007 (or nearest year)

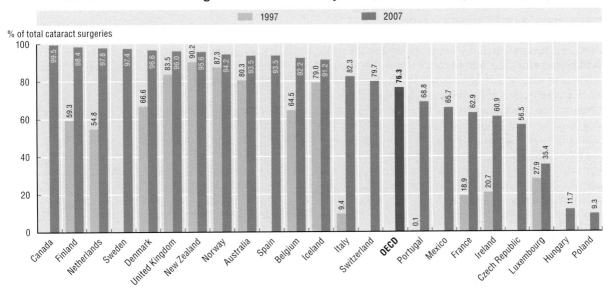

Source: OECD Health Data 2009.

StatLink ⬛🖳 http://dx.doi.org/10.1787/718588776311

The consumption of pharmaceuticals is increasing across OECD countries not only in terms of expenditure (see Indicator 7.4 "Pharmaceutical expenditure"), but also in terms of volume (or quantity) of drugs consumed. One of the factors contributing to the rise in pharmaceutical consumption is the ageing of the population, which leads to growing demand for drugs to treat or at least control different ageing-related diseases. But the trend rise in pharmaceutical consumption is also observed in countries where the population ageing process is less advanced, indicating that other factors such as physicians' prescription habits or the degree of cost-sharing with patients also play a role.

This section provides information on the current level and growth rate in the volume of consumption of four categories of pharmaceuticals: antidiabetics, antidepressants, anticholesterols and antibiotics. The volume of consumption of these drugs is measured through the "defined daily dose" (DDD) unit, which is recommended by the WHO Collaborating Center for Drug Statistics (see the box on "Definition and deviations" below).

There are a lot of variations across countries in the consumption of drugs for the treatment of diabetes, with the consumption in Iceland being almost three times lower than in Finland, Germany or Greece (Figure 4.10.1). These differences can be partly explained by the prevalence of diabetes, which is low in Iceland and relatively high in Germany (see Indicator 1.12). However, some of the top consumers are not countries in which the prevalence of diabetes is high. Between 2000 and 2007, the consumption of antidiabetics increased in all countries. The growth rate was particularly strong in the Slovak Republic (although it started from a low level), the United Kingdom, Denmark, Finland and Iceland. The rise in consumption can be attributed to a rising prevalence of diabetes as well as increases in the proportion of people treated and the average dosages used in treatments (Melander et al., 2006).

Iceland reports the highest level of consumption of antidepressants, followed by Australia and other Nordic countries (Figure 4.10.2). The Slovak Republic, Hungary and the Czech Republic have the lowest levels of consumption, although consumption of antidepressants in these countries has grown rapidly over the past seven years. Germany is an exception with both low levels and slow growth in consumption.

The consumption of anticholesterols ranges from a high of 206 DDDs per 1 000 people per day in Australia to a low of 49 in Germany (Figure 4.10.3). While this might reflect partly differences in the prevalence of high bad cholesterol levels in the population, these differences can also be attributed to differences in clinical guidelines for the control of bad cholesterol. For instance, guidelines in Australia target lower bad cholesterol levels than those in European countries; and differences also exist in target levels within Europe (National Heart Foundation of Australia et al., 2005; Hockley and Gemmill, 2007). Both the epidemiological context (for instance, growing obesity) and increased screening and treatment explain the very rapid growth in the consumption of anticholesterols across all OECD countries for which data are available.

The consumption of antibiotics varies from a low of 9 DDDs per 1 000 people per day in Switzerland to a high of 32 in Greece (Figure 4.10.4). As over-consumption of antibiotics has been acknowledged to create bacterial resistance, many countries have launched in recent years information campaigns targeting physicians and/or patients in order to reduce antibiotic consumption. As a result, consumption has stabilised in many countries and even decreased in some others (such as France, Portugal and the Slovak Republic). By contrast, consumption has risen between 2000 and 2007 in countries that had below-average initial levels of consumption (such as Denmark and Ireland).

Definition and deviations

Defined daily dose (DDD) is defined as the assumed average maintenance dose per day for a drug used on its main indication in adults. DDDs are assigned to each active ingredient(s) in a given therapeutic class by international expert consensus. For instance, the DDD for oral aspirin equals 3 grams, which is the assumed maintenance daily dose to treat pain in adults. DDDs do not necessarily reflect the average daily dose actually used in a given country. DDDs can be aggregated within and across therapeutic classes of the Anatomic-Therapeutic Classification (ATC). For more detail, see www.whocc.no/atcddd.

Data generally refer to out-patient consumption except for the Czech Republic, Finland, Hungary, and Sweden, where data also include hospital consumption. Greek figures may include parallel exports.

4.10.1 Antidiabetics consumption, DDD* per 1 000 people per day, 2000 and 2007 (or nearest year)

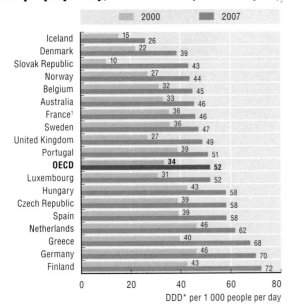

1. Only represent 88% of consumption.

4.10.2 Antidepressants consumption, DDD* per 1 000 people per day, 2000 and 2007 (or nearest year)

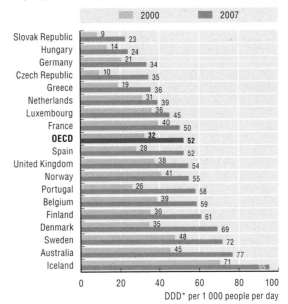

4.10.3 Anticholesterols consumption, DDD* per 1 000 people per day, 2000 and 2007 (or nearest year)

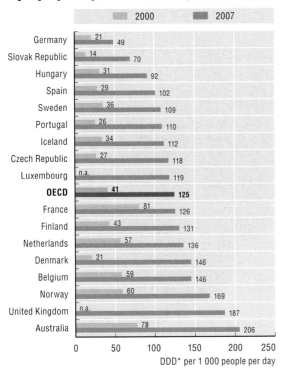

4.10.4 Antibiotics consumption, DDD* per 1 000 people per day, 2000 and 2007 (or nearest year)

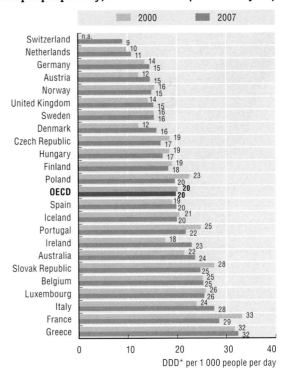

* Defined daily dose.

Source: OECD Health Data 2009.

StatLink ᵐˢᵖ *http://dx.doi.org/10.1787/718618836803*

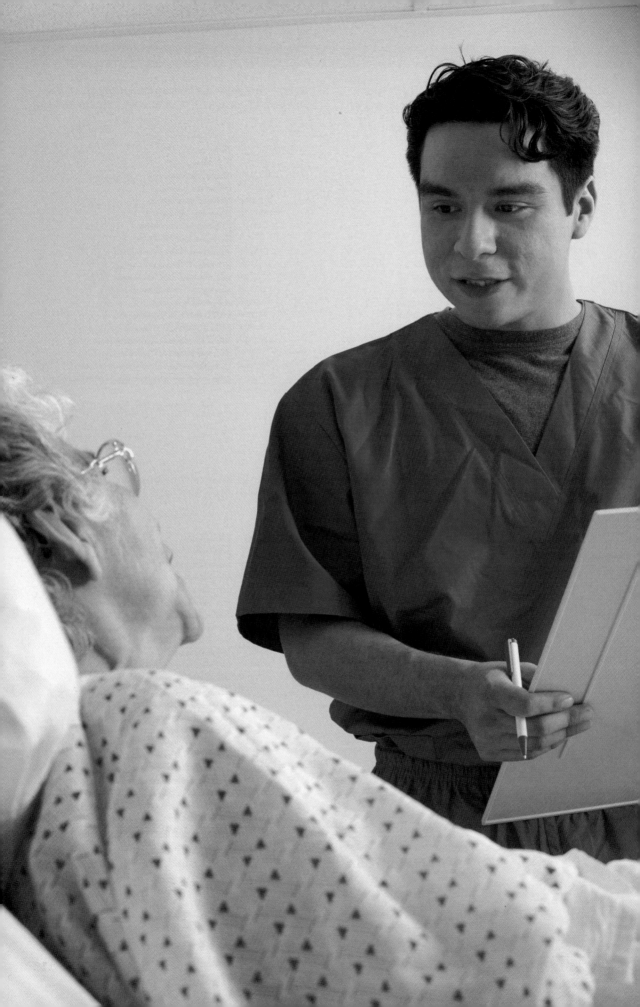

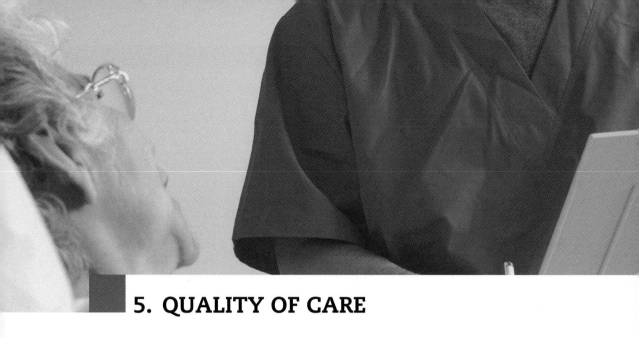

5. QUALITY OF CARE

Introduction

Care for chronic conditions

5.1. Avoidable admissions: respiratory diseases

5.2. Avoidable admissions: diabetes complications

5.3. Avoidable admissions: congestive heart failure, hypertension

Acute care for chronic conditions

5.4. In-hospital mortality following acute myocardial infarction

5.5. In-hospital mortality following stroke

Care for mental disorders

5.6. Unplanned hospital re-admissions for mental disorders

Cancer care

5.7. Screening, survival and mortality for cervical cancer

5.8. Screening, survival and mortality for breast cancer

5.9. Survival and mortality for colorectal cancer

Care for communicable diseases

5.10. Childhood vaccination programmes

5.11. Influenza vaccination for elderly people

Which areas of the health care system are providing value-for-money and which show opportunities for performance improvement? While ongoing national and international efforts, such as the Systems of Health Accounts, are providing better information on health care spending, information on the value that health care services create is still limited. Quality of care, or the degree to which care is delivered in accordance with established standards and optimal outcomes, is one of the key dimensions of value.

Many OECD countries are reporting on quality of care at the national level, whereas other countries are still lacking the data infrastructure to derive such information. Internationally comparable data on quality of care are needed to allow countries to explore underlying factors in the organisation and financing of health care. The OECD's Health Care Quality Indicators project (HCQI) is developing a set of quality indicators at the health care systems level (Mattke et al., 2006; Garcia Armesto et al., 2007). Its approach is to complement and co-ordinate efforts of national and other international bodies. Combined with other initiatives, this effort will offer policy makers and other stakeholders a toolkit to stimulate cross-national learning. All 30 OECD countries, along with five European Union countries that are not member countries, and Singapore, are now participating in the project.

Constructing the toolkit requires three building blocks: a conceptual framework to define the dimensions to be captured; relevant and scientifically sound indicators to reflect performance across those dimensions; and data to implement the selected indicators. Since its inception in 2003, the HCQI project has made significant progress towards assembling the first two components. As discussed in the general introduction of this publication, a conceptual framework has been developed that reflects the shared understanding of countries regarding the key performance dimensions of the health care systems (Kelley and Hurst, 2006). There has been consensus that the project should initially focus on the technical quality of care (i.e. medical effectiveness). Several reviews have also been completed and published to identify suitable indicators for quality of care in areas such as cardiac care, diabetes and mental health.

The main limiting factor, however, remains the availability of data to construct quality indicators, especially at the international level. The limited adoption of electronic health records (EHR) means that the detailed clinical information required for many indicators is often unavailable, restricting the project to indicators that can be derived from more widely available, but less informative administrative data. The lack of use of unique patient identifiers (UPI) in some countries limits the ability to track patients across care settings and institutions and thus the opportunity to capture care pathways longitudinally. Lastly, differences in coding systems and data collection standards hamper the international comparability of indicators.

In spite of those shortcomings, substantial progress has been made. A total of 40 indicators have been adopted, 23 of which are featured in this edition of Health at a Glance. These indicators cover key health care needs, all major health care services, and most major disease areas. New areas covered in this publication, compared with the previous edition of Health at a Glance, are the treatment of chronic conditions in primary care and mental health care. While several coverage gaps remain, such as patient safety and patient experiences, and comparability across countries still needs improvement, the indicators allow policy makers and other stakeholders to begin to draw inferences about relative health care system performance in several key areas. This chapter illustrates the use of HCQI indicators to explore policy questions in the areas of care for chronic conditions, acute exacerbations of chronic diseases, mental disorders, cancer and communicable diseases.

The indicators cover both processes and outcomes of care for a range of conditions (see Table 5.1). The OECD HCQI website, available at www.oecd.org/health/hcqi, provides more information on the sources and methods underlying the data.

5.1 Areas covered by the current set of indicators

	Process measures	Outcome measures
Care for chronic conditions		Avoidable asthma admission rate
		Avoidable chronic obstructive pulmonary disease (COPD) admission rate
		Avoidable diabetes acute complications admission rate
		Avoidable diabetes lower extremity amputation rate
		Avoidable congestive heart failure (CHF) admission rate
		Avoidable hypertension admission rate
Care for acute exacerbations of chronic conditions		Acute Myocardial Infarction (AMI) 30 day case-fatality rate
		Stroke 30 day case-fatality rate
Care for mental disorders		Unplanned schizophrenia re-admission rate
		Unplanned bipolar disorder re-admission rate
Cancer care	Cervical cancer screening rate	Cervical cancer survival rate
	Breast cancer screening rate	Cervical cancer mortality rate
		Breast cancer survival rate
		Breast cancer mortality rate
		Colorectal cancer survival rate
		Colorectal cancer mortality rate
Care for communicable diseases	Rate of childhood vaccination for pertussis	Incidence of hepatitis B
	Rate of childhood vaccination for measles	
	Rate of childhood vaccination for hepatitis B	
	Rate of influenza vaccination for elderly people	

Interpretation and use of the data

The indicators presented in this chapter do not provide a complete assessment of the performance of health care systems with respect to quality of care, as both their comparability and their coverage are limited. Since the last publication of OECD *Health at a Glance* in 2007, efforts have been made to gather data that are as comparable as possible across countries. Improvements include the implementation of clear data quality standards and standard procedures for age and sex adjustment. Confidence intervals have been calculated to identify statistically significant differences between indicator values. Nevertheless, as with other indicators in *OECD Health Data*, differences in definitions, sources and methods remain, and are noted. In particular, additional work on improving comparability and adjusting for differences in patient risk profiles across countries is needed. While the indicators are based on evidence and have been used for research and analysis *within* countries, it is not yet fully understood why they vary *across* countries. The development of further indicators to provide a more comprehensive account of quality remains necessary to allow more robust benchmarking of health care system performance.

The data presented in this chapter should be looked at as raising questions about the quality of care in different countries, rather than providing definitive answers or normative judgments. While information is provided to assure the reader of the importance and scientific soundness of each indicator, the data and findings presented should be considered as a starting point for a better understanding of variations in quality of care and to promote further analysis of different national experiences. Ongoing work under the HCQI project will improve comparability and coverage and offer a more robust view of comparative performance in the future.

5. QUALITY OF CARE

Future priority areas

In line with the established conceptual framework (Kelley and Hurst, 2006; Arah *et al.*, 2006), the OECD HCQI project is seeking to improve and expand the current set of quality of care indicators in the domains of patient safety and responsiveness/patient experiences.

In response to the growing interest in monitoring and improving the safety of medical care (WHO, 2008a; Council of the European Union, 2009), the OECD has been exploring the potential for international comparisons of patient safety using routine hospital administrative data (OECD, 2007c). In 2007, a preliminary study was undertaken among seven OECD member countries to investigate the feasibility of calculating a set of 12 indicators originally published by the United States Agency for Healthcare Research and Quality (AHRQ). Given the encouraging results of this initial study (Drösler *et al.*, 2009a), an extended data collection was undertaken in 2008, involving 16 countries and 15 patient safety indicators (see Table 5.2).

5.2 List of patient safety indicators studied in 2008

Area	Indicator name
Hospital-acquired infections	Decubitus ulcer (PSI 3) Catheter-related bloodstream infections (PSI 7)
Operative and post-operative complications	Complications of anaesthesia (PSI 1) Iatrogenic pneumothorax (PSI 6) Postoperative hip fracture (PSI 8) Postoperative respiratory failure (PSI 11) Postoperative pulmonary embolism (PE) or deep vein thrombosis (DVT) (PSI 12) Postoperative sepsis (PSI 13) Accidental puncture or laceration (PSI 15)
Sentinel events	Foreign body left in during procedure (PSI 5) Transfusion reaction (PSI 16)
Obstetrics	Birth trauma – injury to neonate (PSI 17) Obstetric trauma – vaginal delivery with instrument (PSI 18) Obstetric trauma – vaginal delivery without instrument (PSI 19) Obstetric trauma – caesarean section (PSI 20)

Note: The numbers in brackets refer to the US Agency for Healthcare Research and Quality patient safety indicators.

In order to facilitate comparisons, technical specifications and methods of calculation for these indicators were developed (Drösler, 2008), and the potential impact of national variations in the distribution of age and gender, length of hospital stay and medical and surgical treatment was assessed.

This provided grounds for the OECD to collect seven of the indicators in 2009, namely: catheter-related bloodstream infections, postoperative pulmonary embolism or deep vein thrombosis, postoperative sepsis, accidental puncture or laceration, foreign body left in during procedure, and obstetric trauma after vaginal delivery with or without instrument. A total of 18 countries participated in the third round of data collection in early 2009. However, issues with the completeness and comparability of the underlying data, and caution over the interpretation of the findings means that these indicators are not currently deemed suitable for presentation in this publication.

A detailed technical report on the 2009 data collection and the current state of development of the OECD set of patient safety indicators has been released (Drösler *et al.*, 2009b) and can be downloaded from the OECD website: *www.oecd.org/health/hcqi*. This report identifies the key challenges that need to be addressed to enable meaningful comparisons of patient safety in the future, and foreshadows the ongoing work of the OECD to address data issues and enhance national information infrastructures. In particular, the need for improvements in the routine administrative databases of OECD countries is highlighted. Through the strengthening of secondary diagnoses coding, establishment of condition present-at-admission codes, standardisation of medical procedure codes and further use of unique patient identifiers, international comparability of safety indicators will be significantly enhanced.

In addition to patient safety, the OECD is seeking to address the domain of responsiveness by strengthening the capacity for international measurement of patient experiences of health care. Recent work in collaboration with national experts and international organisations is focussing on the development and application of population-based survey instruments.

The establishment of meaningful indicators in these two priority areas, along with further refinement and development of indicators within existing indicator areas (*e.g.* health promotion, prevention and primary care), will allow a more complete assessment of the quality of care provided through OECD country health systems in the future.

Asthma, a condition characterised by hyper-reactivity and chronic inflammation of the bronchial system, is the most common chronic disease in childhood, with increasing prevalence in recent decades. Childhood asthma prevalence in the United States has doubled to 9% since the 1980s (Moorman *et al.*, 2007). Asthma persists to adulthood in at least 25% of children (Sears *et al.*, 2003). Approximately 30 million people in the European region are affected by asthma (Masoli *et al.*, 2004). ·

Chronic obstructive pulmonary disease (COPD), sometimes referred to as chronic bronchitis, is currently the fourth leading cause of death in the world (WHO, 2006). The most important risk factor is tobacco smoking which causes 80% to 90% of COPD cases. Smokers are ten times more likely to die from COPD than non-smokers (HHS, 2004). Around 11.2 million Americans have manifest COPD and 24 million have evidence of impaired pulmonary function consistent with early stages of COPD (ALA, 2009).

Treatment for asthma with anti-inflammatory agents and bronchodilators in the primary care setting is largely able to prevent exacerbations and, when they occur, most exacerbations can be handled without any need for hospitalisation. High hospital admission rates may therefore be an indication of poor quality of care. Admission rates for asthma have been used to assess quality of care by, for example, the United Kingdom National Health Service, and in the United States National Healthcare Quality Report (AHRQ, 2008b).

While a cure of COPD is not possible, treatment approaches have proven to stabilise patients to avoid the need for hospital admissions (Jadwiga *et al.*, 2007). Innovative approaches, such as the "Hospital at Home" that originated in the United Kingdom, have shown to substantially decrease admission rates and cost (Ram *et al.*, 2004). As much of the responsibility for managing COPD lies with primary care providers, hospital admission rates are a measure of the quality of primary care (AHRQ, 2007b).

Figures 5.1.1 and 5.1.2 show that the age and sex-standardised hospital admission rates for asthma and COPD vary substantially across OECD member countries. While on average 51 out of 100 000 adults are admitted for asthma in a given year, the United States reports over twice this rate (120). Its neighbour Canada

has a much lower rate of 18 admissions. For COPD, variations of similar magnitude are reported. On average, 201 admissions occurred per 100 000 adults in OECD countries, but the rate was as high as 384 in Ireland and as low as 33 in Japan. Austria, for example, reported over three times the rate of neighbouring Switzerland.

Figure 5.1.1 reveals that on average females are about 70% more likely to be admitted to hospital for asthma than males, with the rate for females in the United States being more than double the rates of males. This may be due, at least partly, to the fact that adult asthma prevalence is usually higher in females.

Figure 5.1.3 shows that COPD admission rates are correlated to a certain extent with estimates of COPD prevalence. This analysis points towards the exploration of potential gaps in care in countries with COPD admission rates that are higher than expected based on the reported disease prevalence. A similar correlation was not found between estimates of asthma prevalence and admission rates.

Definition and deviations

The avoidable asthma and COPD hospital admission rate is defined as the number of hospital admissions of people aged 15 years and over per 100 000 population in that age group per year. There is evidence of differences in diagnosis and coding between asthma and COPD across countries which points to limitations in the relative precision of the specific disease rates. Direct comparison of the asthma admission rates between the 2009 and 2007 editions of *Health at a Glance* is cautioned, given the rates for 2009 have been adjusted to take account of differences in the age and sex composition of each country's population and the age cohort has been revised from 18 years to 15 years and over. The prevalence estimates for COPD were self-reported by countries and the validity and comparability of these rates have not been fully assessed.

5.1.1 Asthma admission rates, population aged 15 and over, 2007

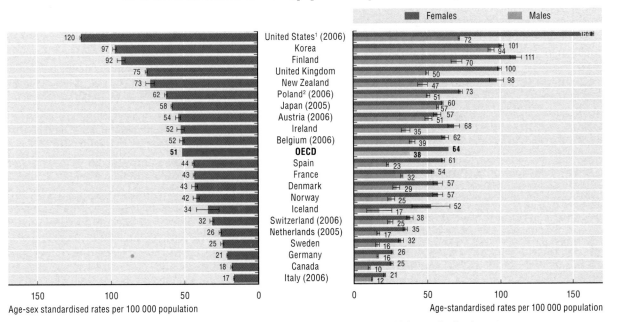

Age-sex standardised rates per 100 000 population

Age-standardised rates per 100 000 population

1. Does not fully exclude day cases.   2. Includes transfers from other hospital units, which marginally elevates rates.

5.1.2 COPD admission rates, population aged 15 and over, 2007

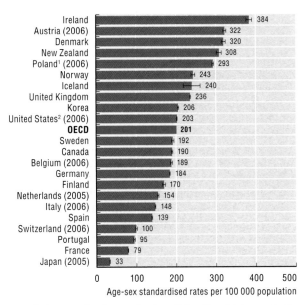

Age-sex standardised rates per 100 000 population

1. Includes transfers from other hospital units, which marginally
   elevates rates.   2. Does not fully exclude day cases.

5.1.3 COPD admission rates and prevalence rates, 2007 (or latest year available)

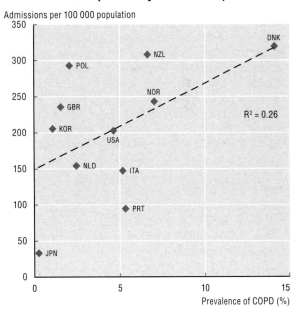

Source: OECD Health Care Quality Indicators Data 2009. Rates are age-sex standardised to 2005 OECD population. 95% confidence intervals are represented by ⊢—⊣ .

StatLink ᴍᴤᴾ http://dx.doi.org/10.1787/718683484730

5.2. Avoidable admissions: diabetes complications

Driven by the rise in obesity rates, diabetes has become one of the most important public health challenges of the 21st century. Over 150 million adults are affected worldwide, with the number expected to double in the next 25 years (King et al., 1998; IDF, 2006). Across OECD countries, prevalence is estimated to be more than 6% of the population aged 20-79 years in 2010 and ranges from less than 5% in Iceland, Norway and the United Kingdom to more than 10% in Mexico and the United States, (see Indicator 1.12 "Diabetes prevalence and incidence"). Diabetes is the leading cause of blindness in industrialised countries and the most common cause of end-stage renal disease in the United States, Europe, and Japan. Individuals with type II diabetes have a two-to-four times greater risk of cardiovascular disease (Haffner, 2000).

There is evidence that lifestyle changes such as weight loss and increased physical activity can prevent diabetes in high-risk individuals (Tuomilehto et al., 2001). Better glycaemic control limits organ damage and vascular complications over time (Diabetes Control and Complications Trial Research Group, 1996). Empirical data, however, reveals that such practices are underutilised (McGlynn et al., 2003).

Hospital admissions for lower extremity (or limb) amputation reflect the quality of long-term diabetes treatment. Non-traumatic amputations are 15 times more frequent in diabetic patients than in the general population and 80% of amputations could be prevented, according to WHO estimates (Ollendorf et al., 1998; WHO, 2005). Appropriate diet, exercise and drug treatment combined with proper foot care can reduce the risk of lower extremity amputation. Since most related services are delivered or ordered by primary care providers, both admissions for acute diabetic complications and lower extremity amputations are suitable measures of the quality of primary care.

Figure 5.2.1 reveals that many countries have rates of diabetes-related lower extremity amputation close to the OECD average of 15 amputations per 100 000 population, but the United States has more than twice that rate with 36 admissions. Korea and Austria, on the other hand, have only about half the average admission rate.

Admission rates for amputations are higher for men, even though diabetes is slightly more prevalent in women. Figure 5.2.1 reveals that diabetic males are admitted for lower extremity amputations at a rate nearly threefold that of females. This likely reflects the higher rates of vascular risk factors other than diabetes in men (AHRQ, 2009).

Figure 5.2.2 illustrates that the United States has the highest admission rate for acute diabetic complications, with almost 60 admissions per 100 000 population or almost three times the OECD average rate of 21. The rate is below ten admissions in New Zealand and the Netherlands. Some countries have explicit targets to improve diabetes treatment at the primary care level. For instance, New Zealand has established a service target to increase the percentage of people with diabetes who attend a free health check and have satisfactory diabetes management (Ministry of Health, 2007).

Figure 5.2.3 shows that amputation rates are not strongly correlated with estimates of diabetes prevalence, indicating that the underlying rate of diabetes does not explain most of the variation in amputation rates. This, together with the magnitude of the variations for both acute complications and amputations, indicates that further investigation of systems of care is warranted.

Definition and deviations

Avoidable diabetes acute complication and lower extremity amputation hospital admission rates are defined as the number of hospital admissions of people aged 15 years and over per 100 000 population in that age group per year. Coding practices for primary and secondary diagnoses between countries might affect indicator rates. The rates have been adjusted to take account of differences in the age and sex composition of each country's population. The definition of the lower extremity amputation indicator includes amputation of the foot and toes in addition to more major amputations, such as above ankle, through knee and up to hip amputations. Minor amputations of the toe and foot do not necessarily indicate poor quality of care, as they may be carried out to prevent major amputations. In addition, given some minor amputations can be performed in certain primary care settings, clinical practices between countries might also affect indicator rates. Since definition rely on specific procedure codes, different classification systems in use across countries may impact on the comparability of the data.

5.2.1 Diabetes lower extremity amputation rates, population aged 15 and over, 2007

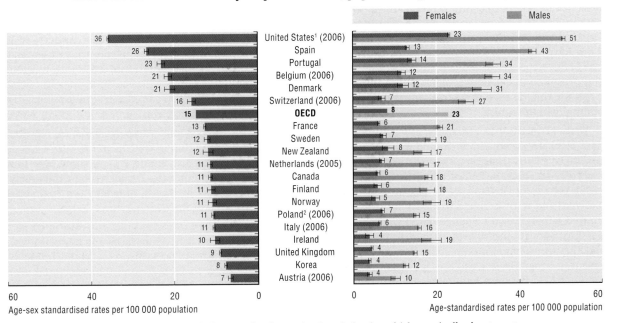

Females   Males

	Females	Males
United States[1] (2006)	36	23 — 51
Spain	26	13 — 43
Portugal	23	14 — 34
Belgium (2006)	21	12 — 34
Denmark	21	12 — 31
Switzerland (2006)	16	7 — 27
OECD	**15**	**8 — 23**
France	13	6 — 21
Sweden	12	7 — 19
New Zealand	12	8 — 17
Netherlands (2005)	11	7 — 17
Canada	11	6 — 18
Finland	11	6 — 18
Norway	11	5 — 19
Poland[2] (2006)	11	7 — 15
Italy (2006)	11	6 — 16
Ireland	10	4 — 19
United Kingdom	9	4 — 15
Korea	8	4 — 12
Austria (2006)	7	4 — 10

60   40   20   0   0   20   40   60
Age-sex standardised rates per 100 000 population   Age-standardised rates per 100 000 population

1. Does not fully exclude day cases. 2. Includes transfers from other hospital units, which marginally elevates rates.

5.2.2 Diabetes acute complications admission rates, population aged 15 and over, 2007

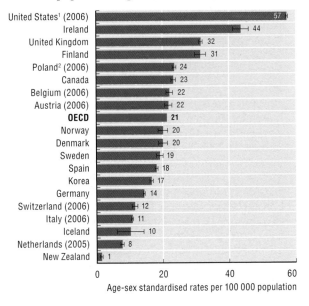

United States[1] (2006)	57
Ireland	44
United Kingdom	32
Finland	31
Poland[2] (2006)	24
Canada	23
Belgium (2006)	22
Austria (2006)	22
OECD	**21**
Norway	20
Denmark	20
Sweden	19
Spain	18
Korea	17
Germany	14
Switzerland (2006)	12
Italy (2006)	11
Iceland	10
Netherlands (2005)	8
New Zealand	1

0   20   40   60
Age-sex standardised rates per 100 000 population

1. Does not fully exclude day cases. 2. Includes transfers from other hospital units, which marginally elevates ates.

5.2.3 Diabetes lower extremity amputation rates and prevalence of diabetes, 2007

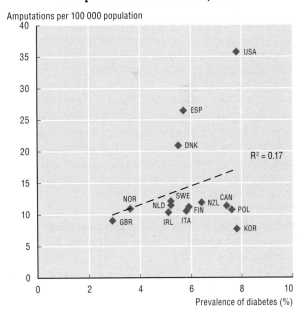

Amputations per 100 000 population

$R^2 = 0.17$

Prevalence of diabetes (%)

Source: OECD Health Care Quality Indicators Data 2009. Rates are age-sex standardised to 2005 OECD population. Diabetes prevalence (aged 20-79 years) are from the International Diabetes Federation (2006). 95% confidence intervals are represented by ⊢⊣.

StatLink 🔗 http://dx.doi.org/10.1787/718688035313

5.3. Avoidable admissions: congestive heart failure, hypertension

Congestive heart failure (CHF), the inability of the heart to provide adequate circulation, is a severe condition with prevalence estimates of around 5% in Portugal and Denmark, and 3% in England (Ceia *et al.*, 2002; Raymond *et al.*, 2003; Davies *et al.*, 2001). As the risk of developing heart failure increases with age and the presence of cardiovascular disease, prevalence rates for this disease are expected to increase substantially in the future.

Outpatient medical treatment with vasodilators and beta-blockers, combined with fluid management and controlled exercise, has been shown to improve survival rates of heart failure (SOLVD Investigators, 1991; CIBIS-II, 1999). Data from the Euro Heart Survey II on patients hospitalised with congestive heart failure showed limited adherence to evidence-based treatment, suggesting room to improve outpatient management of those patients (Komajda *et al.*, 2003). Data from the same research programme also revealed that one quarter (24%) of CHF patients had been re-admitted within 12 weeks of discharge and 14% of patients died between admission and 12 weeks follow-up (Cleland *et al.*, 2003). Given the high rate of re-admissions, even small improvements in care can have a substantial impact on cost and patient quality of life (Lee *et al.*, 2004).

Hypertension or high blood pressure is the most common chronic condition of adult populations. Its global prevalence in the adult population was estimated to be over 26% in 2000 (Kearney *et al.*, 2005). In itself, hypertension rarely causes symptoms but it is a risk factor for a variety of cardiovascular diseases, such as stroke, heart failure, and renal insufficiency. It is also associated with other cardiovascular risk factors, such as diabetes and hypercholesterolemia.

Admissions with a primary diagnosis of hypertension typically indicate hypertensive crises, a condition characterised by very high blood pressure with high risk of acute complications such as heart failure or hemorrhagic stroke. However, hypertension admissions are largely avoidable and are an indicator for the quality of primary care (Tisdalea *et al.*, 2004).

Figure 5.3.1 shows that Poland and the United States record the highest CHF admission rates with over 440 admissions per 100 000 population, about twice the OECD average of 234. The United Kingdom and Korea, on the other hand, have only about a fourth of the highest level of admissions. The gender gap is particularly large for the Nordic countries of Iceland, Denmark and Sweden where the male rate is about double the female rate, whereas on average in OECD countries admissions for men are only about 50% more frequent than for women.

Just over 80 admissions for hypertension are reported per 100 000 population in OECD countries on average (Figure 5.3.2), but Austria and Poland show over four and three times this rate, respectively. Conversely, countries such as the United Kingdom and Spain only report a fraction of the average rate.

The overall use of admitted patient care is closely correlated with admission rates for hypertension (Figure 5.3.3). About two-thirds of the variation in admission rates for hypertension is associated with the variation for admissions for any cause. Countries like Austria have both above-average rates for hospital admissions for any cause and for hypertension, whereas countries like Canada and Spain have low rates for both.

Definition and deviations

The avoidable CHF and hypertension hospital admission rates are defined as the number of hospital admissions of people aged 15 years and over per 100 000 population in that age group per year. The rates have been adjusted to take account of differences in the age and sex composition of each country's population. Given the technical definition of these indicators includes the specification of procedure codes, the different classification systems in use across countries may impact on the comparability of the data.

5.3.1 CHF admission rates, population aged 15 and over, 2007

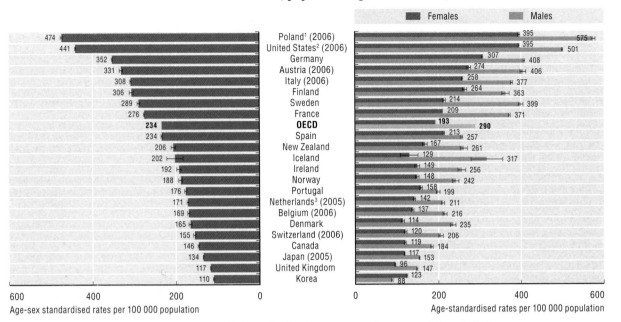

Age-sex standardised rates per 100 000 population

Age-standardised rates per 100 000 population

1. Includes transfers from other hospital units, which marginally elevates rates.   2. Does not fully exclude day cases.
3. Includes admissions for additional diagnosis codes, which marginally elevates rates.

5.3.2 Hypertension admission rates, population aged 15 and over, 2007

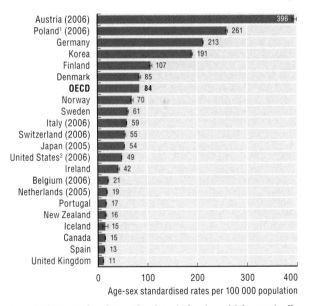

Age-sex standardised rates per 100 000 population

1. Includes transfers from other hospital units, which marginally elevates rates.   2. Does not fully exclude day cases.

5.3.3 Hypertension admission rates and total admission rates, 2007 (or latest year available)

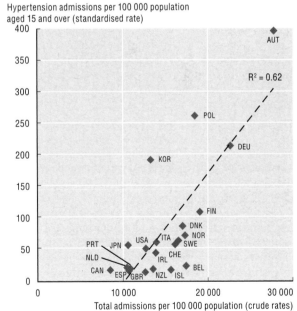

Source: OECD Health Care Quality Indicators Data 2009. Rates are age-sex standardised to 2005 OECD population. 95% confidence intervals are represented by ⊢──┤.

StatLink ⊞⊠┛ http://dx.doi.org/10.1787/718721288366

Although coronary artery disease (CAD) remains the leading cause of death in most industrialised countries, mortality rates have declined since the 1970s (see Indicator 1.4 "Mortality from heart disease and stroke"). Much of the reduction can be attributed to lower mortality from acute myocardial infarction (AMI), due to better treatment in the acute phase. Care for AMI has changed dramatically in recent decades, with the introduction of coronary care units in the 1960s (Khush et al., 2005) and with the advent of treatment aimed at rapidly restoring coronary blood flow in the 1980s (Gil et al., 1999). This success is all the more remarkable as data suggest that the incidence of AMI has not declined (Goldberg et al., 1999; Parikh et al., 2009). However, numerous studies have shown that a considerable proportion of AMI patients fail to receive evidence-based care (Eagle et al., 2005). AMI accounts for about half of the deaths from CAD, with the cost of care for CAD accounting for as much as 10% of health care expenditures in industrialised countries (OECD, 2003a).

Evidence links the processes of care for AMI, such as thrombolysis and early treatment with aspirin and beta-blockers, to survival improvements, suggesting that the case-fatality rate for AMI is a suitable measure of quality of care (Davies et al., 2001). Given the variety of services and system devices that need to be mobilised to provide care for this illness, the AMI case-fatality rate is regarded as a good outcome measure of acute care quality. Currently, AMI case-fatality rates have been used for hospital benchmarking by the United States Agency for Healthcare Research and Quality (Davies et al., 2001) and the United Kingdom's National Health Service. It has also been employed for international comparisons by the OECD Ageing-Related Diseases Project (OECD, 2003a) and the WHO Monica Project (Tunstall-Pedoe, 2003).

Figure 5.4.1 shows crude and age-sex standardised in-hospital case-fatality rates within 30 days of admission for AMI. The average standardised rate is just below 5%, with the rate being the highest in Korea (8.1%) and the lowest in Iceland (2.1%) and Sweden (2.9%). Other Nordic countries (Finland, Norway and Denmark) are also below the average. Differences in hospital transfers, average length of stay and emergency retrieval times can influence reported rates. In countries with highly specialised emergency services, more patients reach the hospital alive but can ultimately not be stabilised and die within hours of admission. In other countries, unstable cardiac patients are commonly transferred to tertiary care centres, possibly biasing case-fatality rates downward, if the transfer is recorded as a live discharge. Case-fatality rates for women with AMI are typically higher, but the difference is not statistically significant for all countries. This reflects the fact that, while coronary artery disease is much more common in men, it is usually more severe in women.

Figure 5.4.2 shows that case-fatality rates for AMI are decreasing over time in all reporting OECD countries, with the majority recording statistically significant reductions between 2003 and 2007. In Canada and other countries, improvements in AMI case fatality rates reflect advances in treatment such as the increased rates and timeliness of reperfusion therapy, which seeks to restore blood flow to that part of the heart muscle damaged during heart attack (Fox et al., 2007 and Tu et al., 2009).

Definition and deviations

The in-hospital case-fatality rate following AMI is defined as the number of people who die within 30 days of being admitted (including same day admissions) to hospital with an AMI. Ideally, rates would be based on individual patients, however, not all countries have the ability to track patients in and out of hospital, across hospitals or even within the same hospital because they do not currently use a unique patient identifier. Therefore, this indicator is based on individual hospital admissions and restricted to mortality within the same hospital. Differences in practices in discharging and transferring patients may influence the findings.

Both crude and age-sex standardised rates are presented. Standardised rates adjusts for differences in age (45+ years) and sex and facilitate more meaningful international comparisons. Crude rates are likely to be more meaningful for internal consideration by individual countries and enable a more direct comparison with the crude rates presented for this indicator in *Health at a Glance 2007*.

5.4.1 In-hospital case-fatality rates within 30 days after admission for AMI, 2007

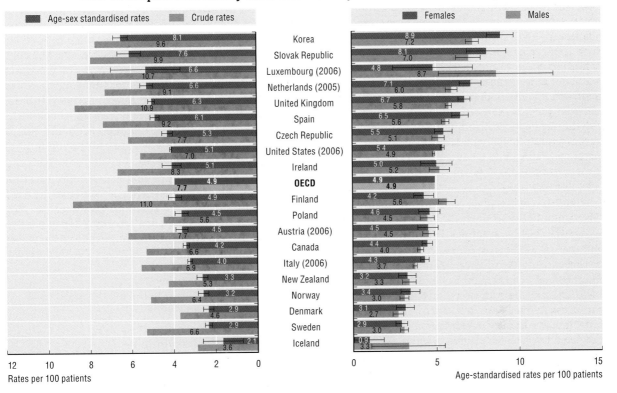

5.4.2 Reduction in in-hospital case-fatality rates within 30 days after admission for AMI, 2003-07 (or nearest year available)

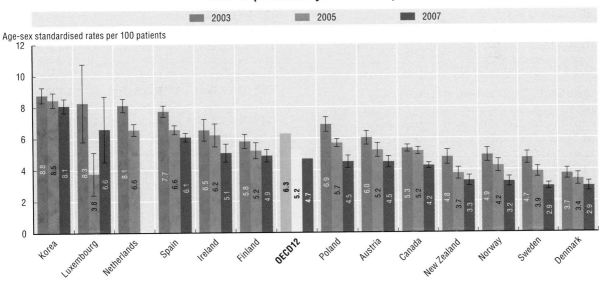

Source: OECD Health Care Quality Indicators Data 2009. Rates are age-sex standardised to 2005 OECD population (45+). 95% confidence intervals are represented by ⊢─┤ .

StatLink ᵃᵐˢᵖ *http://dx.doi.org/10.1787/718746461517*

Stroke remains the third most common cause of death and disability in industrialised countries (WHO, 2002). Estimates suggest that it accounts for 2-4% of health care expenditure and also for significant costs outside of the health care system due to its impact on disability (OECD, 2003a). In ischemic stroke, representing about 85% of cases, the blood supply to a part of the brain is interrupted, leading to a necrosis of the affected part. In hemorrhagic stroke, rupture of a blood vessel causes bleeding into the brain, usually causing more widespread damage.

Treatment for ischemic stroke has changed dramatically over the last decade. Until the 1990s, it was largely accepted that the damage to the brain was irreversible and treatment focused on prevention of complications and rehabilitation. But following the spectacular improvements in AMI survival rates that were achieved with early thrombolysis, clinical trials (starting in Japan in the early 1990s) demonstrated clear benefits of thrombolytic treatment for ischemic stroke (Mori et al., 1992). Dedicated stroke units, modelled after the very successful Cardiac Care Unit, were introduced in many countries, particularly in Nordic countries, to facilitate timely and aggressive diagnosis and therapy of stroke victims. A recent meta-analysis of 18 studies showed that stroke units achieved about 20% better survival than usual care (Seenan et al., 2007).

Large randomised clinical trials in the United States (e.g. NINDS, 1995) and Europe (e.g. Hacke et al., 1995) have unambiguously demonstrated the impact of thrombolytic therapy for ischemic stroke on survival and disability. However, adoption of this practice is met with resistance due to factors related to the organisation of health services (Wardlaw et al., 2003; Wahlgren et al., 2007). Stroke case-fatality rates have been used for hospital benchmarking within and between countries (OECD, 2003; Sarti et al., 2003).

While the average standardised case fatality rate for ischemic stroke is 5%, there is nearly a fourfold difference between the highest rate in the United Kingdom (9.0%) and the lowest rates in Iceland (2.3%) and Korea (2.4%) (Figure 5.5.1). Figure 5.5.2 shows the age and sex standardised and crude rates for hemorrhagic stroke. The average rate is 19.8%, about four times greater than the rate for patients with ischemic stroke, which reflects the more severe effects of intracranial bleeding. There is more than a threefold difference in reported rates between Luxembourg (30.3%) and the Slovak Republic (29.3%), and Finland (9.5%).

Figure 5.5.3 illustrates that case-fatality rates for ischemic and hemorrhagic stroke are correlated; that is, countries that achieve better survival for one type of stroke tend to also do well for the other type. Given the initial steps of care for stroke patients are similar, this suggests that systems-based factors play a role in explaining the differences across by countries. For example, a cluster of Nordic countries (Finland, Sweden, Norway, Denmark and Iceland) lie below the OECD average for both ischemic and hemorrhagic stroke. These countries have been at the forefront of establishing dedicated stroke units in hospitals.

Figure 5.5.4 demonstrates that case-fatality rates for both hemorrhagic and ischemic stroke have declined by around 15% across OECD countries between 2002 and 2007, with all countries recording a decrease in both forms of stroke. This suggests widespread improvement in the quality of care.

Definition and deviations

The in-hospital case-fatality rate following ischemic and hemorrhagic stroke is defined as the number of people who die within 30 days of being admitted (including same day admissions) to hospital. Ideally, rates would be based on individual patients, however, not all countries have the ability to track patients in and out of hospital, across hospitals or even within the same hospital given they do not currently use a unique patient identifier. Therefore, this indicator is based on unique hospital admissions and restricted to mortality within the same hospital. Differences in practices in discharging and transferring patients may influence the findings.

Both crude and age and sex standardised rates are presented. Standardised rates adjusts for differences in age (45+ years) and sex and facilitate more meaningful international comparisons. Crude rates are likely to be more meaningful for internal consideration by individual countries and enable a more direct comparison with the crude rates presented for this indicator in Health at a Glance 2007.

5.5.1 In-hospital case-fatality rates within 30 days after admission for ischemic stroke, 2007

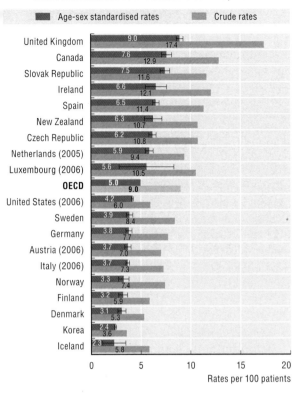

5.5.2 In-hospital case-fatality rates within 30 days after admission for hemorrhagic stroke, 2007

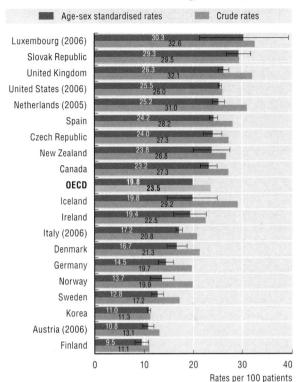

5.5.3 In-hospital case-fatality rates within 30 days after admission for ischemic and hemorrhagic stroke, 2007

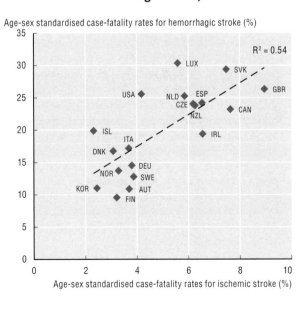

5.5.4 Reduction in in-hospital case-fatality within 30 days after admission for stroke, 2002-07

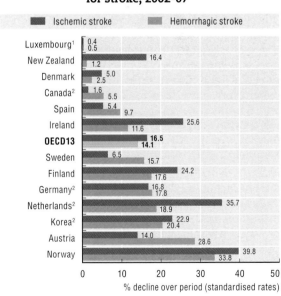

1. Based on 2002-03 to 2006.   2. Based on 3-year period only.

Source: OECD Health Care Quality Indicators Data 2009. Rates are age-sex standardised to 2005 OECD population (45+). 95% confidence intervals are represented by ⊢−⊣.

StatLink ⊓§⌐ *http://dx.doi.org/10.1787/718755164764*

The burden of mental illness is substantial. Schizophrenia and bipolar disorder are among the top ten causes of years lost due to disability at the global level (WHO, 2001).

Mental health care has become a policy priority in many OECD countries, coinciding with dramatic changes in the delivery of mental health services, especially for severe disorders such as schizophrenia and bipolar disorder. Starting with de-institutionalisation in the 1970s, care has shifted from large psychiatric hospitals towards community-based care. Paradoxically, the shift has made it harder to track mental health care at the population level, as few countries have a health information infrastructure suitable for following patients across a variety of delivery settings.

Unplanned hospital re-admission rates are commonly used as an indicator of insufficient care co-ordination following an inpatient stay for psychiatric disorders. Longer lengths of stay, appropriate discharge planning, and follow-up visits after discharge contribute to fewer re-admissions, indicating that re-admission rates reflect the overall functioning of mental health services rather than the quality of hospital care (Lien, 2002). Thirty-day hospital re-admission rates are part of mental health performance monitoring systems in many countries, such as the Care Quality Commission in the United Kingdom and the National Mental Health Performance Monitoring System in the United States.

Figure 5.6.1 shows the variation in unplanned re-admission rates for schizophrenia, with Nordic countries at the higher end and the Slovak Republic, the United Kingdom, Spain and Italy at the lower end. The pattern of re-admission rates for bipolar disorders (Figure 5.6.2) is similar, with the Nordic countries well above average. Most countries have similar rates for men and women, however, male patients with schizophrenia have higher rates in Italy while female patients are more likely to be re-admitted in Canada and Denmark. Regarding bipolar disorder patients, women have higher re-admission rates in Finland, Sweden, Ireland, Canada and Belgium. These numbers may reflect differences in care seeking behaviours or management related to a patient's gender.

Supply factors such as the availability of hospitals beds (psychiatric and total), and the profile of in-patient facilities (percentage of in-patient care provided in psychiatric hospitals, general acute hospitals or residential facilities) cannot explain the variation in re-admission rates. The average length of stay for patients with schizophrenia or bipolar disorder does not seem to be associated with variations in re-admission rates. Anecdotal evidence suggests that different approaches to crisis management might play a part. For example, some countries with lower re-admission rates, such as the United Kingdom, Spain and Italy, use community-based "crisis teams" to stabilise patients on an outpatient basis. Other countries with high rates, such as Finland and Denmark, use interval care protocols to place unstable patients into hospital care for short periods. While there is broad consensus that community-based care is preferable to in-hospital care where possible, in certain countries the practice seems to be shifting towards supplementing or substituting community-based devices with in-hospital care. In the absence of a comparable measure of outcomes across countries, the benefits of this alternative approach are difficult to assess. The enhancement of mental health related information systems will be necessary to make this type of comparative information readily available.

Definition and deviations

The indicator is defined as the number of unplanned re-admissions per 100 patients with a diagnosis of schizophrenia and bipolar disorder per year. The denominator is comprised of all patients with at least one admission during the year for the condition. A re-admission is considered unplanned when the patient is admitted for any mental disorder to the same hospital within 30 days of discharge. Same-day admissions (less than 24 hours) are excluded.

The absence of unique patient identifiers in many countries does not allow the tracking of patients across facilities. Rates are therefore biased downwards as re-admissions to a different facility cannot be observed. However, the eight countries which were able to estimate re-admission rates to the same or other hospitals, show that rates based on the two different specifications were closely correlated and ranking of countries was similar, suggesting that re-admissions to the same hospital can be used as a valid approximation.

5.6.1 Unplanned schizophrenia re-admissions to the same hospital, 2007

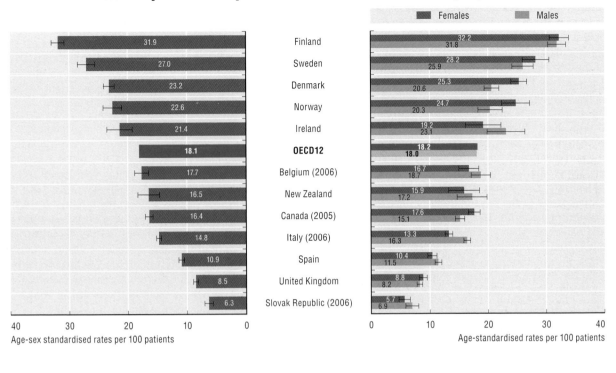

Age-sex standardised rates per 100 patients

Age-standardised rates per 100 patients

5.6.2 Unplanned bipolar disorder re-admissions to the same hospital, 2007

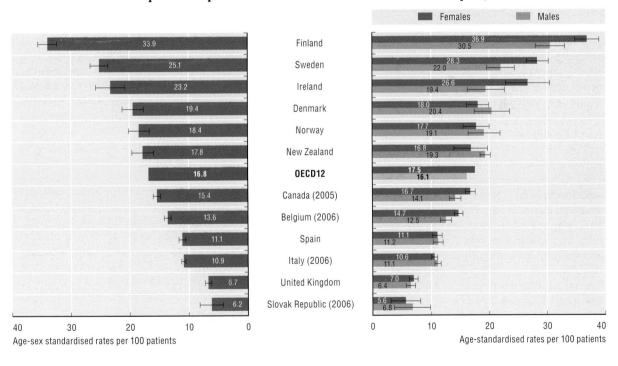

Age-sex standardised rates per 100 patients

Age-standardised rates per 100 patients

Source: OECD Health Care Quality Indicators Data 2009. Rates are age-sex standardised to 2005 OECD population. 95% confidence intervals are represented by ⊢─┤ .

StatLink ⌐╗╝ http://dx.doi.org/10.1787/718800331705

Cervical cancer is largely preventable. Screening by regular pelvic exam and pap smears can identify premalignant lesions, which can be effectively treated before the occurrence of the cancer. Regular screening also increases the probability of diagnosing early stages of the cancer and improving survival (Gatta et al., 1998). The Council of the European Union and the European Commission promote population based cancer screening programmes among member States (European Union, 2003; European Commission, 2008c). OECD countries have instituted screening programmes, but the periodicity and target groups vary. In addition, the discovery that cervical cancer is caused by sexual transmission of certain forms of the Human Papilloma Virus has led to the development of promising cancer preventing vaccines (Harper et al., 2006). The efficacy and safety of those vaccines is now well established, but debates about cost-effectiveness and the implications of vaccination programmes for teenagers for a sexually transmitted disease continue in a number of countries (Huang, 2008).

Three indicators are presented to reflect variation in cervical cancer care across OECD countries: cervical cancer screening rates in women aged 20-69 years, five-year relative survival rates, and mortality rates for cervical cancer.

Relative survival rates are commonly used to track progress in treating a disease over time. They reflect both how early the cancer was detected and the effectiveness of the treatment provided. Mortality rates alone are not sufficient to draw timely inferences about quality of care, because current mortality rates reflect the effect of cancer care in past years and changes in incidence. Survival rates have been used to compare European countries in the EUROCARE study, in comparisons between European countries and the United States (Gatta et al., 2000), and in national reporting activities in many countries.

Screening rates vary widely across OECD countries with the United States and the United Kingdom achieving coverage of around 80% of the target population (Figure 5.7.1). Some countries with very low screening rates, like Japan and Hungary, have no uniform national screening programme; the low rates reflect local programmes or opportunistic screening. The data indicates that screening rates in several countries slightly declined between 2000 and 2006.

Nearly all countries recorded five-year relative survival rates above 60% for the period 2002-07. The rates ranged from 76.5% in Korea to 50.1% in Poland (Figure 5.7.2). Over the periods 1997-2002 and 2002-07, the five-year relative rates improved in most coun-

tries, although in most instances the increase is not statistically significant.

Figure 5.7.3 shows that mortality rates for cervical cancer declined for most OECD countries between 1995 and 2005, with larger improvements for many countries with initially higher rates, such as Mexico and several central and eastern European countries.

Definition and deviations

Screening rates for cervical cancer reflect the proportion of patients who are eligible for a screening test and actually receive the test. As policies regarding screening periodicity differ across countries, the rates are based on each country's specific policy. An important consideration is that some countries ascertain screening based on surveys and others based on encounter data, which may influence the results. If a country has an organised screening programme, but women receive care outside the programme, rates may be underreported. Survey-based results may also underestimate the rates due to recall bias.

Relative cancer survival rates reflect the proportion of patients with a certain type of cancer who are still alive after a specified time period (commonly five years) compared to those still alive in absence of the disease. Relative survival rates capture the excess mortality that can be attributed to the diagnosis. To illustrate, a relative survival rate of 80% does not mean that 80% of the cancer patients are still alive after five years, but that 80% of the patients that were expected to be alive after five years, given their age at diagnosis, are in fact still alive. All the survival rates presented here have been age-standardised using the International Cancer Survival Standard (ICSS) population. Data reported in Health at a Glance 2007 were not age standardised, therefore, rates presented in this edition cannot be compared with those from the previous edition. The survival rates are not adjusted for tumour stage at diagnosis, hampering assessment of the relative impact of early detection and better treatment.

See Indicator 1.5 "Mortality from cancer" for definition, source and methodology underlying the cancer mortality rates.

5.7.1 Cervival cancer screening, percentage of women screened aged 20-69, 2000 to 2006 (or nearest year)

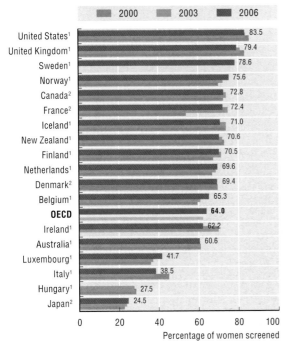

Legend: 2000, 2003, 2006

United States[1]	83.5
United Kingdom[1]	79.4
Sweden[1]	78.6
Norway[1]	75.6
Canada[2]	72.8
France[2]	72.4
Iceland[1]	71.0
New Zealand[1]	70.6
Finland[1]	70.5
Netherlands[1]	69.6
Denmark[2]	69.4
Belgium[1]	65.3
OECD	**64.0**
Ireland[1]	62.2
Australia[1]	60.6
Luxembourg[1]	41.7
Italy[1]	38.5
Hungary[1]	27.5
Japan[2]	24.5

Percentage of women screened

5.7.2 Cervical cancer five-year relative survival rate, 1997-2002 and 2002-07 (or nearest period)

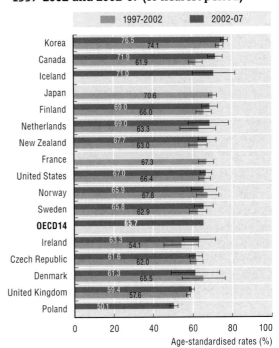

Legend: 1997-2002, 2002-07

Country	1997-2002	2002-07
Korea	76.5	74.1
Canada	71.9	61.9
Iceland	71.0	
Japan		70.6
Finland	69.0	66.0
Netherlands	69.0	63.3
New Zealand	67.7	63.0
France		67.3
United States	67.0	66.4
Norway	65.9	67.8
Sweden	65.8	62.9
OECD14	65.7	
Ireland	63.3	54.1
Czech Republic	61.6	62.0
Denmark	61.3	65.5
United Kingdom	59.4	57.6
Poland	50.1	

Age-standardised rates (%)

1. Programme.   2. Survey.

5.7.3 Cervical cancer mortality, females, 1995 to 2005 (or nearest year)

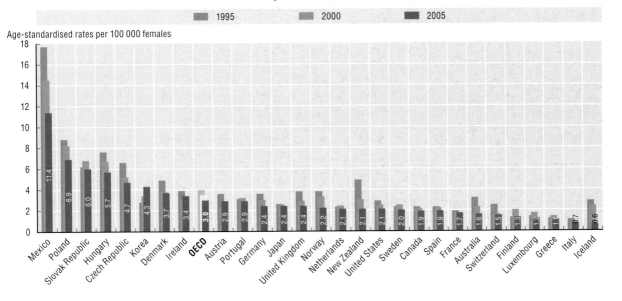

Age-standardised rates per 100 000 females

Legend: 1995, 2000, 2005

Mexico 11.4, Poland 6.9, Slovak Republic 6.0, Hungary 5.7, Czech Republic 4.7, Korea 4.3, Denmark 3.7, Ireland 3.4, OECD 3.0, Austria 2.9, Portugal 2.9, Germany 2.4, Japan 2.4, United Kingdom 2.4, Norway 2.2, Netherlands 2.1, New Zealand 2.1, United States 2.1, Sweden 2.0, Canada 1.9, Spain 1.9, France 1.7, Australia 1.6, Switzerland 1.5, Finland 1.3, Luxembourg 1.2, Greece 1.1, Italy 0.7, Iceland 0.6

Source: OECD Health Care Quality Indicators Data 2009. Survival rates are age standardised to the International Cancer Survival Standards population. *OECD Health Data 2009* (cancer screening; mortality data extracted from the WHO Mortality Database and age standardised to the 1980 OECD population). 95% confidence intervals are represented by ⊢⊣ in the relevant figures.

StatLink ⟨⟨⟨ http://dx.doi.org/10.1787/718838163700

Breast cancer is the most common form of cancer in women, with a lifetime incidence of about 11% and a lifetime mortality rate of about 3% in the United States (Feuer *et al.*, 2003). One in nine women will acquire breast cancer at some point in their life and one in thirty will die from the disease. Overall spending for breast cancer care typically amounts to about 0.5-0.6% of total health care expenditure (OECD, 2003a).

The combination of public health interventions and improved medical technology has contributed to substantial improvements in survival rates for breast cancer. Greater awareness of the disease and the promotion of self-examination and screening mammography (European Union, 2003; European Commission, 2006) have led to the detection of the disease at earlier stages. Technological improvements, such as the introduction of combined breast conserving surgery with radiation therapy and routine adjuvant chemotherapy treatment, have increased survival as well as the quality of life of survivors (Mauri *et al.*, 2008).

Three indicators are presented to reflect the variation in breast cancer care across OECD countries: mammography screening rates in women 50-69 years, relative survival rates, and mortality rates for breast cancer. Clinical studies have demonstrated the effectiveness of breast cancer screening and treatment in improving survival. Even though the optimal frequency of screening and the age-group to target are still the subject of debate, most countries have adopted screening programmes. For example, EU guidelines (European Commission, 2006) promote a target screening rate of at least 75% of eligible women in European countries.

Resources and patterns for breast cancer treatment vary substantially across OECD countries, leading to an interest in comparing survival and mortality rates (OECD, 2003a). Breast cancer survival rates have been used to compare countries in the EUROCARE study (Sant *et al.*, 2009), and in the CONCORD study (Coleman *et al.*, 2008) among other studies.

In the Netherlands and Finland, close to 90% of women aged 50-69 years are screened annually, but only around 20% in the Slovak Republic and Japan (Figure 5.8.1). Some countries with very low screening rates, like Japan, have no national screening programme; the low rates reflect opportunistic screening or local programmes. Some countries which had low rates in 2000, such as the Czech and Slovak Republics, showed substantial increases by 2006, whereas some countries with already high rates experienced declines, including the United States, Finland and Norway.

Many OECD countries have survival rates of over 80%, with rates as high as 90% for the United States (Figure 5.8.2). The United States reports the highest survival rate for women diagnosed in 2002 and a screening rate for that year which is among the highest in the OECD. Given the effect of early detection through screening requires several years before it is manifest, the impact of the decrease in the United States mammography rates between 2000 and 2006 will remain uncertain until survival rates for future years become available.

Figure 5.8.2 shows that relative five-year breast cancer survival rates have improved slightly in almost all countries between 1997-2002 and 2002-07, even though changes are usually not statistically significant. However, data from European countries over a longer time period confirm that five-year survival rates for breast cancer have increased over recent years and particularly in eastern European countries that historically had lower survival rates (Verdecchia *et al.*, 2007).

Figure 5.8.3 illustrates that breast cancer mortality rates are declining in most OECD countries. Korea and Japan are the exceptions, though the changes are small and mortality levels continue to be the lowest among OECD countries. Conversely, improvements are substantial for countries that had higher levels in 1995, like the Netherlands, the United Kingdom, Ireland and Denmark.

Definition and deviations

Mammography screening rates reflect the proportion of eligible women patients who are actually screened. As policies regarding target age groups and screening periodicity differ across countries, the rates are based on each country's specific policy. Some countries ascertain screening based on surveys and others based on encounter data, and this may influence results. If a country has an organised screening programme, but women receive care outside of the programme, rates may be underreported. Survey-based results may also underestimate rates due to recall bias.

Survival rates and mortality rates are defined in Indicator 5.7 "Cervical cancer".

5.8.1 Mammography screening, percentage of women aged 50-69 screened, 2000 to 2006 (or nearest year available)

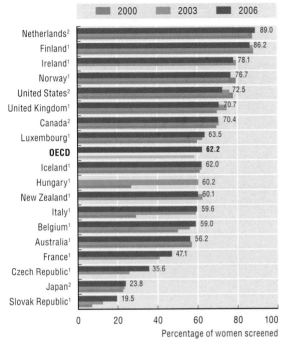

1. Programme. 2. Survey.

5.8.2 Breast cancer five-year relative survival rate, 1997-2002 and 2002-07 (or nearest year available)

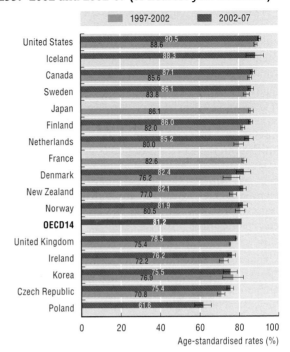

5.8.3 Breast cancer mortality, females, 1995 to 2005 (or nearest year available)

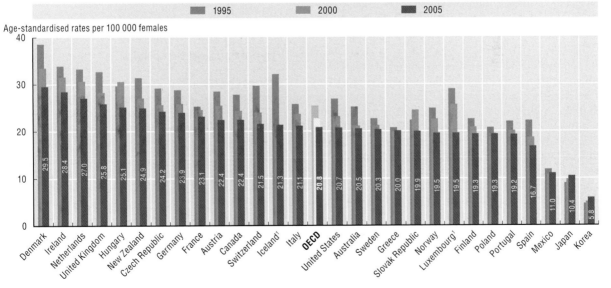

1. Rates for Iceland and Luxembourg are based on a three-year average.

Source: OECD Health Care Quality Indicators Data 2009. Survival rates are age standardised to the International Cancer Survival Standards population. *OECD Health Data 2009* (cancer screening; mortality data extracted from WHO Mortality Database and age standardised to 1980 OECD population). 95% confidence intervals are represented by ⊢⊣ in the relevant figures.

StatLink 📊 http://dx.doi.org/10.1787/718845186853

5.9. Survival and mortality for colorectal cancer

Colorectal cancer is the third most common form of cancer in both women (after breast and lung cancer) and men (after prostate and lung cancer). It is estimated that approximately USD 8.4 billion is spent in the United States each year on the treatment of colorectal cancer (Brown *et al.*, 2002). Advances in diagnosis and treatment have increased survival over the last decades.

Evidence exists that demonstrates the clinical benefit of screening with routine colonoscopy and stool tests for occult blood (USPSTF, 2008) and various treatment modalities, such as surgery (Govindarajan *et al.*, 2006) and chemotherapy (CCCG, 2000), even for advanced stages of the disease. The same literature suggests that screening and treatment options are not sufficiently utilised. However, although organised screening programmes are being piloted in several OECD countries, data on screening rates for colorectal cancer are not yet available at an international level.

Variation in outcomes for patients with colorectal cancer is captured by five-year relative survival rates and mortality rates. Colorectal cancer survival rates have been used to compare European countries in the EUROCARE study (Sant *et al.*, 2009), to compare countries around the world in the CONCORD study (Coleman *et al.*, 2008), and in many national reporting activities.

Figure 5.9.1 presents the most recent five-year relative survival rates for patient with colorectal cancer. Japan has the highest relative survival rate of 67%, followed by Iceland and the United States with rates above 65%. Poland has the lowest rate with 38%, followed by the Czech Republic and the United Kingdom, Ireland and Denmark.

All countries show improvement in survival rates over time (Figure 5.9.2), although the increase is often not statistically significant. The United States which had the highest survival rate of 62.5% for patients diagnosed in 1997 improved to 65.5% for those diagnosed in 2000. The Czech Republic improved from 41% to 47% for the periods 1997-2002 and 2001-06.

Historical data from France shows that the five-year survival rate between 1976 and 1988 increased from 33% to 55%, which is attributed to a higher resection rate with lower post-operative mortality, earlier diagnosis and increasing use of chemotherapy (Faivre-Finn *et al.*, 2002). These findings are consistent with results from other European countries (Sant *et al.*, 2009) and the United States (SEER, 2009). Recent data from the EUROCARE project showed that survival for colorectal cancer continued to increase in Europe, and in particular in eastern European countries (Verdecchia *et al.*, 2007).

Mortality trends from colorectal cancer for the period from 1995 and 2005 are shown in Figure 5.9.3. Most countries experienced a decrease in mortality for colorectal cancer in these ten years. While Korea's rates have increased markedly over time, these rates are still among the lowest in OECD countries. The rapid introduction of western-type diet is a possible explanation for this increase. As Figure 5.9.2 illustrates, Korea has achieved a significant increase in relative survival rates over recent years, indicating that the health care system is addressing this new challenge. Central and eastern European countries tend to have higher mortality rates with no clear geographic pattern emerging for the other OECD countries. Countries with high relative survival rates, like Japan and the United States also have below-average mortality rates, which supports the hypothesis that the differences in relative survival reflect better cancer care.

Definition and deviations

Survival rates and mortality rates are defined in Indicator 5.7 "Cervical cancer" and vary from the ICD 10 definition of colorectal cancer employed in *Health at a Glance 2007* by also including anal cancer.

5.9.1 Colorectal cancer, five-year relative survival rate, total and male/female, latest period

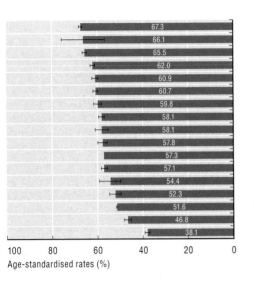

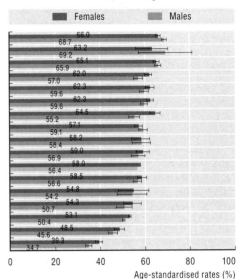

Country	Total
Japan (1999-2004)	67.3
Iceland (2003-08)	66.1
United States (2000-05)	65.5
Finland (2002-07)	62.0
New Zealand (2002-07)	60.9
Canada (2000-05)	60.7
Sweden (2003-08)	59.8
Korea (2001-06)	58.1
Netherlands (2001-06)	58.1
Norway (2001-06)	57.8
OECD	57.3
France (1997-2002)	57.1
Denmark (2002-07)	54.4
Ireland (2001-06)	52.3
United Kingdom (2002-07)	51.6
Czech Republic (2001-06)	46.8
Poland (2002-07)	38.1

Females / Males

Age-standardised rates (%)

5.9.2 Colorectal cancer, five-year relative survival rate, 1997-2002 and 2002-07 (or nearest period)

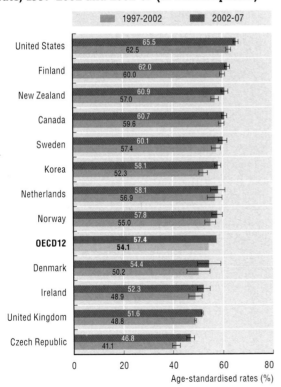

1997-2002 / 2002-07

Country	2002-07	1997-2002
United States	65.5	62.5
Finland	62.0	60.0
New Zealand	60.9	57.0
Canada	60.7	59.6
Sweden	60.1	57.4
Korea	58.1	52.3
Netherlands	58.1	56.9
Norway	57.8	55.0
OECD12	**57.4**	**54.1**
Denmark	54.4	50.2
Ireland	52.3	48.9
United Kingdom	51.6	48.8
Czech Republic	46.8	41.1

Age-standardised rates (%)

5.9.3 Colorectal cancer mortality, 1995 to 2005 (or nearest year)

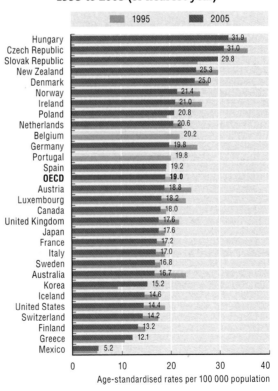

1995 / 2005

Country	2005
Hungary	31.9
Czech Republic	31.0
Slovak Republic	29.8
New Zealand	25.3
Denmark	25.0
Norway	21.4
Ireland	21.0
Poland	20.8
Netherlands	20.6
Belgium	20.2
Germany	19.8
Portugal	19.8
Spain	19.2
OECD	**19.0**
Austria	18.8
Luxembourg	18.2
Canada	18.0
United Kingdom	17.6
Japan	17.6
France	17.2
Italy	17.0
Sweden	16.8
Australia	16.7
Korea	15.2
Iceland	14.6
United States	14.4
Switzerland	14.2
Finland	13.2
Greece	12.1
Mexico	5.2

Age-standardised rates per 100 000 population

Source: OECD Health Care Quality Indicators Data 2009. Survival rates are age standardised to the International Cancer Survival Standards population. *OECD Health Data 2009* (mortality data extracted from WHO Mortality Database and age standardised to 1980 OECD population). 95% confidence intervals are represented by ⊢─┤ in the relevant figures.

StatLink ⟨⟨⟨ *http://dx.doi.org/10.1787/720027814582*

5.10. Childhood vaccination programmes

Childhood vaccination continues to be one of the most cost-effective health policy interventions. All OECD countries or, in some cases, sub-national jurisdictions have established vaccination programmes based on their interpretation of the risks and benefits of each vaccine.

Vaccination against pertussis (often administered in connection with vaccination against diphtheria and tetanus) and measles is part of almost all programmes, and reviews of the evidence supporting the efficacy of vaccines against these diseases have concluded that the respective vaccines are safe and highly effective. In Europe, the gradual uptake of the measles vaccine has meant that measles incidence is around ten times less than the rate of the early 1990s.

A vaccination for hepatitis B has been available since 1982 and is considered to be 95% effective in preventing infection and its chronic consequences, such as cirrhosis and liver cancer. In 2004, it was estimated that over 350 million people were chronically infected with the hepatitis B virus worldwide and at risk of serious illness and death (WHO, 2009a).

In 2007, more than 170 countries had already begun to follow the WHO recommendation to incorporate hepatitis B vaccine as an integral part of their national infant immunisation programmes. In countries with low levels of hepatitis B (e.g. Australia, New Zealand, northern and western Europe and North America) the WHO indicates that routine hepatitis B vaccination should still be given high priority given a high proportion of chronic infections are acquired during early childhood (WHO, 2004a).

Figures 5.10.1 and 5.10.2 demonstrate that the overall vaccination of children against measles and pertussis (including diphtheria and tetanus) is high in OECD countries. On average more than 90% of 2-year-old children receive the recommended measles and pertussis vaccination, and rates for all countries are above 75%.

Figure 5.10.3 shows the average percentage of children aged 2 years who are vaccinated for hepatitis B across countries with national programmes is over 95%. A number of countries do not currently require children to be vaccinated by age 2, or do not have routine programmes and consequently the rates for these countries are significantly lower than the other countries. For example, in Denmark and Sweden, vaccination against hepatitis B is not an obligatory part of their vaccination programmes, and is only recommended to specific risk groups. While Canada implemented universal hepatitis B vaccination for adolescents, not all provinces and territories offer programmes in early infancy (Public Health Agency of Canada, 2009; and Mackie et al., 2009). In France, hepatitis B vaccination remains controversial, given ongoing speculation over possible side effects.

Figure 5.10.4 indicates that the incidence of hepatitis B in the majority of OECD countries is low, at less than two per 100 000 population. Only Austria, Turkey and Iceland have rates well above the OECD average of 2.5 per 100 000 population, and fall into the high-incidence category, based on WHO criteria (WHO, 2004a).

Definition and deviations

Vaccination rates reflect the percentage of children at either age 1 or 2 that receives the respective vaccination in the recommended timeframe. Childhood vaccination policies differ slightly across countries. Thus, these indicators are based on the actual policy in a given country. Some countries administer combination vaccines (e.g. DTP for diphtheria, tetanus and pertussis) while others administer the vaccinations separately. Variations in rate may exist where the tetanus vaccination rate has been provided in place of the pertussis rate, although these are estimated to be less than 0.5%. Some countries ascertain vaccinations based on surveys and others based on encounter data, which may influence the results.

5.10.1 Vaccination rates for pertussis, children aged 2, 2007 (or latest year available)

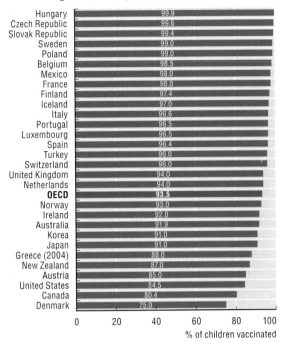

% of children vaccinated

Country	Value
Hungary	99.9
Czech Republic	99.6
Slovak Republic	99.4
Sweden	99.0
Poland	99.0
Belgium	98.5
Mexico	98.0
France	98.0
Finland	97.4
Iceland	97.0
Italy	96.6
Portugal	96.5
Luxembourg	96.5
Spain	96.4
Turkey	96.0
Switzerland	96.0
United Kingdom	94.0
Netherlands	94.0
OECD	**93.5**
Norway	93.0
Ireland	92.0
Australia	91.9
Korea	91.0
Japan	91.0
Greece (2004)	88.0
New Zealand	87.0
Austria	85.0
United States	84.5
Canada	80.4
Denmark	75.0

5.10.2 Vaccination rates for measles, children aged 2, 2007 (or latest year available)

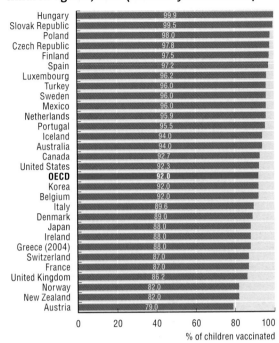

% of children vaccinated

Country	Value
Hungary	99.9
Slovak Republic	99.5
Poland	98.0
Czech Republic	97.8
Finland	97.5
Spain	97.2
Luxembourg	96.2
Turkey	96.0
Sweden	96.0
Mexico	96.0
Netherlands	95.9
Portugal	95.5
Iceland	94.0
Australia	94.0
Canada	92.7
United States	92.3
OECD	**92.0**
Korea	92.0
Belgium	92.0
Italy	89.6
Denmark	89.0
Japan	88.0
Ireland	88.0
Greece (2004)	88.0
Switzerland	87.0
France	87.0
United Kingdom	86.2
Norway	82.0
New Zealand	82.0
Austria	79.0

5.10.3 Vaccination rates for hepatitis B, children aged 2, 2007 (or latest year available)

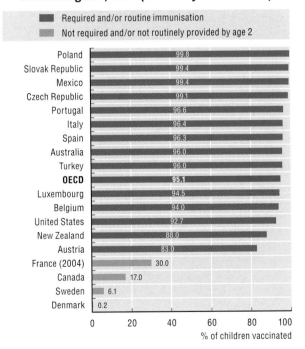

- ▉ Required and/or routine immunisation
- ▉ Not required and/or not routinely provided by age 2

% of children vaccinated

Country	Value
Poland	99.8
Slovak Republic	99.4
Mexico	99.4
Czech Republic	99.1
Portugal	96.6
Italy	96.4
Spain	96.3
Australia	96.0
Turkey	96.0
OECD	**95.1**
Luxembourg	94.5
Belgium	94.0
United States	92.7
New Zealand	88.0
Austria	83.0
France (2004)	30.0
Canada	17.0
Sweden	6.1
Denmark	0.2

5.10.4 Incidence of hepatitis B, total population, 2007 (or latest year available)

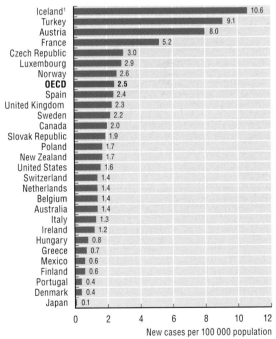

New cases per 100 000 population

Country	Value
Iceland[1]	10.6
Turkey	9.1
Austria	8.0
France	5.2
Czech Republic	3.0
Luxembourg	2.9
Norway	2.6
OECD	**2.5**
Spain	2.4
United Kingdom	2.3
Sweden	2.2
Canada	2.0
Slovak Republic	1.9
Poland	1.7
New Zealand	1.7
United States	1.6
Switzerland	1.4
Netherlands	1.4
Belgium	1.4
Australia	1.4
Italy	1.3
Ireland	1.2
Hungary	0.8
Greece	0.7
Mexico	0.6
Finland	0.6
Portugal	0.4
Denmark	0.4
Japan	0.1

Note: OECD average only includes countries with required or routine immunisation.

1. Based on a three-year average.

Source: OECD Health Data 2009.

StatLink ᵐˢ┻ *http://dx.doi.org/10.1787/720037281182*

5.11. Influenza vaccination for elderly people

Influenza is a common infectious disease worldwide and affects persons of all ages. For example, on average, between 5% and 20% of the population in the United States contracts influenza each year (CDC, 2009b). Most people with the illness recover quickly, but elderly people and those with chronic medical conditions are at higher risk for complications and even death. Between 1979 and 2001, on average, influenza accounted for more than 200 000 hospitalisations and 36 000 deaths per year in the United States (CDC, 2009b). The impact of influenza on the employed population is substantial, even though most influenza morbidity and mortality occurs among the elderly and those with chronic conditions (Keech et al., 1998). In Europe, influenza accounts for around 10% of sickness absence from work, while the cost of lost productivity in France and Germany has been estimated to be in the range of USD 9.3 billion to 14.1 billion per year (Szucs, 2004).

Immunisation against seasonal influenza (or flu) for older people has become increasingly widespread in OECD countries over the past decade. Influenza vaccination for older people and patients with chronic conditions is strongly recommended in Europe, the United States and other countries (Nicholson et al., 1995).

Figure 5.11.1 shows that in 2007 the average percentage of the population aged 65 years and over who were vaccinated for influenza is 56%. However, a wide variation in vaccination rates exists, ranging from 24% in the Czech Republic to 78% in Australia.

Figure 5.11.2 indicates that while the OECD average increased markedly between 1998 and 2003, the average rate remained relatively stable between 2003 and 2007. From 2003, some countries marginally increased their coverage whereas others reduced their coverage, most notably some of the countries which were already below the OECD average, such as the Slovak Republic and Hungary.

A number of factors have contributed to the current levels in influenza immunisation rates in OECD countries, including greater acceptance of preventative health services by patients and practitioners, improved public health insurance coverage for vaccines and wider delivery by health care providers other than physicians (Singleton et al., 2000). A number of barriers need to be overcome in some countries if they wish to further increase their cover-

age rates. For example, possible reasons put forward for the relatively low vaccination rates in Austria include poor public awareness, inadequate insurance coverage of related costs and lack of consensus within the Austrian medical profession about the importance of vaccination (Kunze et al., 2007).

Particularly virulent strains of the virus, similar to the H5N1 avian influenza subtype, can cause pandemics with a much wider impact than seasonal influenza. The impact of influenza not just on the health of people but also on economic activity has been demonstrated again by the H1N1 epidemic (also referred to as "swine flu"). Although the economic impact of the H1N1 epidemic has not been fully assessed, the World Bank estimated in 2008 that a severe flu pandemic could cost the global economy up to 4.8% of world domestic product (Burns et al., 2008).

The WHO reports that vaccines are one of the most valuable ways to protect people during influenza epidemics and pandemics. Other measures include anti-viral and other drugs, social distancing and personal hygiene. Although established national infrastructure and processes for seasonal vaccination programmes can signal an enhanced preparedness to respond to an influenza outbreak, the best scientific evidence suggests that the seasonal influenza vaccines that are routinely provided across OECD countries offer little or no protection against influenza A (H1N1). The development and distribution of effective vaccines takes more than six months (WHO, 2009b).

Definition and deviations

Influenza vaccination rate refers to the number of people aged 65 and older who have received an annual influenza vaccination, divided by the total number of people over 65 years of age. The main limitation in terms of data comparability arises from the use of different data sources, whether survey or programme, which are susceptible to different types of errors and biases. For example, data from population surveys may reflect some variation due to recall errors and irregularity of administration.

5.11.1 Influenza vaccination coverage, population aged 65 and over, 2007 (or latest year available)

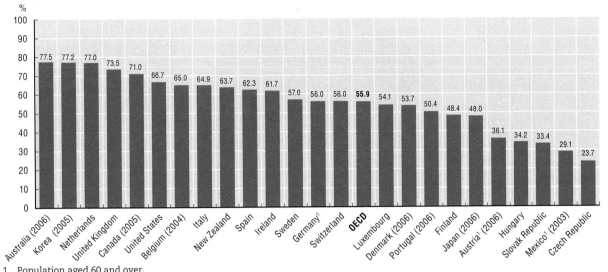

1. Population aged 60 and over.

5.11.2 Vaccination rates for influenza, population aged 65 and over, 1998-2007 (or nearest year available)

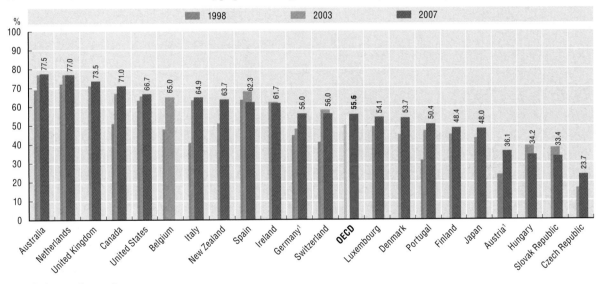

1. Population aged 60 and over.

Source: OECD Health Data 2009.

StatLink http://dx.doi.org/10.1787/720105217254

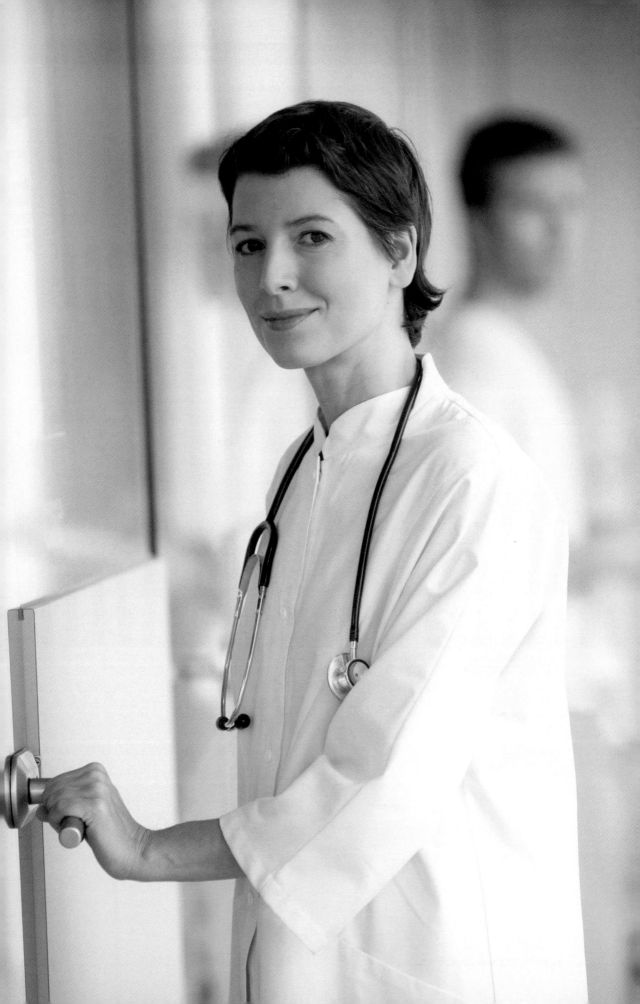

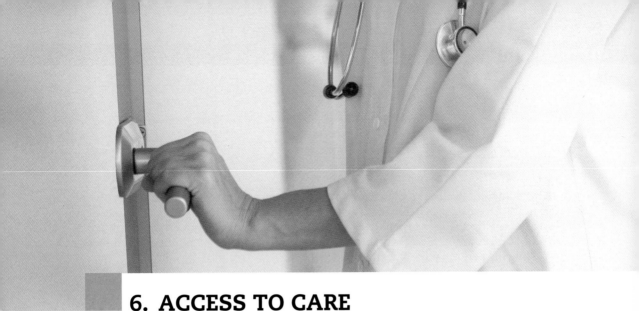

6. ACCESS TO CARE

Introduction

This edition of *Health at a Glance* introduces a chapter on access to health care, building on recent OECD work in this area (de Looper and Lafortune, 2009). Ensuring adequate access to essential health care services on the basis of individual need is an important health policy goal in all OECD countries. Monitoring health care access is, therefore, an important dimension in assessing the performance of health care systems.

Health care access can be defined as an individual's ability to obtain appropriate health care services (Academy Health, 2004). Potential barriers to access include: financial barriers (not being able to afford the costs of care), geographic barriers (not having enough health care providers in a particular geographic area or excessive travelling distance to providers), racial, cultural and information barriers (including language problems) and barriers in terms of timely access (excessive waiting time to see providers).

The indicators presented in this chapter relate only to financial and geographic barriers to health care. In most cases, the information does not cover all countries and some indicators require more recent data. Further work will be needed to provide a more complete and up-to-date picture in future editions, through collaboration with national experts and data correspondents. No information is provided on waiting times for different services. The OECD is planning to update the earlier information that was reported on waiting times for a set of elective surgeries (Siciliani and Hurst, 2003), as well as to broaden the data collection effort to measure waiting for other health services. This work is expected to enrich the content of this chapter in future editions of *Health at a Glance*.

In looking at financial barriers to care, the indicators that are presented focus on inequalities by income groups. However, the availability of comparable data for some indicators is limited. For instance, it was only possible to gather data on the share of out-of-pocket health expenditure by income groups (Indicator 6.3) for a minority of countries.

This chapter looks at access to both medical and dental care. It begins with a review of the available data on self-reported unmet needs for medical and dental care (Indicator 6.1), as a broad measure of access problems. It is a subjective measure, in the sense that it reflects the opinion of individuals on their needs and the degree to which they are met. Individual responses to survey questions on unmet care needs may be affected by recent policy changes and by cultural factors. It is therefore important to look at results of self-reported unmet care needs along with other indicators of access, such as the degree of public or private health insurance coverage (Indicator 6.2) and the burden of out-of-pocket payments (Indicator 6.3) in order to obtain a more complete assessment of health care access in different countries.

Geographic access to care is measured by the "density" of doctors in different regions within each country (Indicator 6.4). A frequent problem in many OECD countries is that doctors tend to concentrate in urban centres, creating access problems for people living in rural and remote areas. However, it has only been possible to collect specific data on the number of doctors practising in urban and rural areas for a few countries, and even within that group of countries, there are differences in how urban and rural regions are defined.

One approach to measure inequalities in access is to measure inequalities in the actual use of health services for different population groups, taking into account differences in need, where applicable and possible. The last three indicators in this chapter look at the use of doctors and dentists and in recommended screening for cancer by socio-economic status (mainly by income group). The indicators rely on data published in an earlier OECD study (van Doorslaer *et al.*, 2004), as well as data gathered by WHO (WHO, 2008b). Much of the information on utilisation rates, however, is derived from studies published some time ago, although efforts to collect more recent data for certain countries generally confirm earlier findings.

More generally, the data used for the indicators are sourced from *OECD Health Data*, and other relevant national and cross-national data surveys and collections.

Most OECD countries aim to provide equal access to health care for people in equal need. One method of gauging equity of access to services is through assessing reports of unmet needs for health care for some reason. The problems that patients report in getting care when they are ill or injured often reflect significant barriers to care.

Some common reasons that people give for unmet care include excessive treatment costs, long waiting times in order to receive care, not being able to take time off work or caring for children or others, or that they had to travel too far to receive care. The different levels of self-reported unmet care needs *across* countries could be due to differences in survey questions, socio-cultural reasons, and also because of reactions to current national health care debates. However, these factors should play a lesser role in explaining any differences in unmet care needs among different population groups *within* each country. It is also important to look at indicators of self-reported unmet care needs in conjunction with other indicators of potential barriers to access, such as the extent of health insurance coverage and out-of-pocket payments (Indicators 6.2 and 6.3).

In most OECD countries, a majority of the population report no unmet care needs. However, in a European survey undertaken in 2007, a significant proportion of the population in some countries reported having unmet needs for medical care during the previous year. Generally, more women than men reported not getting the care they needed, as did people in low-income groups.

Three possible reasons that might lead to access problems are presented in Figure 6.1.1. In almost all countries, the most common reason given for unmet medical care is treatment cost. This was especially so in Portugal, Poland, Italy and Greece, and persons in the lowest income quintile were most affected. Waiting times were an issue for respondents in Italy, Poland, Sweden and the United Kingdom, and affected both higher and lower income persons. Travelling distance did not feature as a major problem, except in Norway, where one-third of those indicating that they had an unmet care need said that it was because of the distance they had to travel to receive care.

A larger proportion of the population reports unmet needs for dental care than for medical care. Poland (7.5%), Italy (6.7%) and Iceland (6.5%) reported the highest rates in 2007 (Figure 6.1.2). Large inequalities in unmet dental care needs were evident between high and low income groups in Iceland, Greece, Portugal and Denmark, as well as in Belgium, although in the latter country, average levels of unmet dental care were low.

Inequalities in self-reported unmet medical and dental care needs are also evident in non-European countries, based on the results of another multi-country survey (Figures 6.1.3 and 6.1.4). Again, foregone care due to costs is more prevalent among lower income groups for a number of different treatments. There are large differences in the size of these inequalities across countries, as shown by much lower levels in the Netherlands and United Kingdom than in the United States. In the United States, more than half the adult population with below-average incomes reported having some type of unmet care need due to cost in 2007 (Commonwealth Fund, 2008). Those adults with below-average incomes who have health insurance report significantly less access problems due to cost than do their uninsured counterparts (Blendon *et al.*, 2002).

Definition and deviations

Questions on unmet health care needs are a feature of a number of national and cross-national health interview surveys, including the European Union Statistics on Income and Living Conditions survey (EU-SILC) and the international health policy surveys conducted by the Commonwealth Fund. No single survey or study on unmet care needs has been conducted across all OECD countries.

In order to determine unmet medical care, individuals are typically asked questions to determine whether there was a time in the previous 12 months when they felt they needed health care services but did not receive them, followed by a question to determine why the need for care was unmet. Common reasons given include that care was too expensive, the travelling distance to receive care was too far, or that the waiting list for care was too long.

Information on both unmet care and socio-economic status are derived from the same survey, although specific questions and answers, along with age groups surveyed and the measures used to grade socio-economic status can vary across surveys and countries. Cultural factors and changes to national health care systems may also affect attitudes to unmet care. Caution is therefore needed in comparing the magnitude of inequalities across countries.

6.1.1 Unmet need for a medical examination, selected reasons by income quintile, European countries, 2007

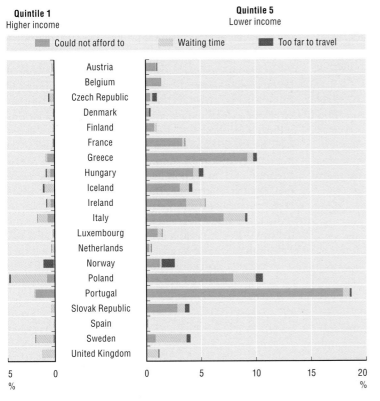

6.1.2 Unmet need for a dental examination, by income quintile, European countries, 2007

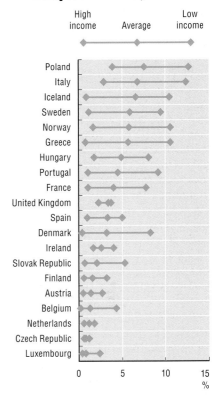

Source: EU-SILC.

6.1.3 Unmet care need[1] due to costs in seven OECD countries, by income group, 2007

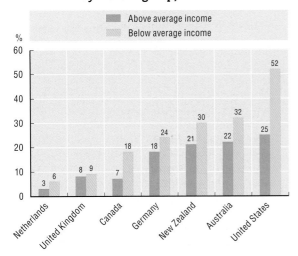

6.1.4 Unmet need for a dental examination due to costs in five OECD countries, by income group, 2004

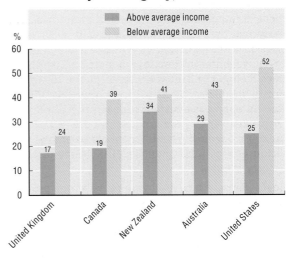

1. Did not get medical care, missed medical test, treatment or follow-up, did not fill prescription or missed doses.

Source: Commonwealth Fund (2008).

Source: Davis *et al.* (2007).

StatLink http://dx.doi.org/10.1787/720134365423

Health care coverage promotes access to medical goods and services, providing financial security against unexpected or serious illness, as well as improved accessibility to treatments and services (OECD, 2004c). Total population coverage (both public and private) is, however, an imperfect indicator of accessibility, since this depends on the services included and on the degree of cost-sharing applied to those services.

By 2007, most OECD countries had achieved universal or near universal coverage of health care costs for a "core" set of services (Figure 6.2.1). Generally, services such as dental care and pharmaceutical drugs are partially covered, but there are a number of countries where these services must be purchased separately (see Annex Table A.5).

Three OECD countries do not have universal health coverage. In Mexico, only half of the population was covered by public health insurance in 2002. The "Seguro Popular" voluntary health insurance scheme was introduced in 2004 to provide coverage for the poor and uninsured, and has grown rapidly, so that by 2007 over 80% of the population were covered. The Mexican government aims to achieve universal coverage by 2011. Public coverage in Turkey was available for only two-thirds of the population in 2003, although recent legislation has introduced universal coverage (OECD and World Bank, 2008).

In the United States, coverage is provided mainly through private health insurance, and 58% of the total population had this in 2007. Publically financed coverage insured 27% of the total population (the elderly, people with low income or with disabilities), leaving 15% of the population (45 million people under 65 years of age) without health coverage. Of these, more than one-half cite the cost of premiums as the reason for their lack of coverage (NCHS, 2009). Recent rises in the proportion of uninsured persons have been attributed to employers, particularly smaller ones, being less likely to offer coverage to workers, and to the increasing cost of premiums (OECD, 2008c). The problem of persistent uninsurance is seen as a major barrier to receiving health care, and more broadly, to reducing health inequalities among population groups (AHRQ, 2008a; HHS Office of Health Reform, 2009).

Basic primary health coverage, whether provided through public or private insurance, generally covers a defined "basket" of benefits, in many cases with cost-sharing. In some countries, additional health coverage can be purchased through private insurance. Among 26 OECD countries, seven (Netherlands, France, Belgium, Canada, United States, Luxembourg and Ireland) report private coverage for over half of the population in 2007 (Figure 6.2.2). In the Netherlands, the government implemented a mandatory universal health insurance scheme in 2006, with regulated competition across private insurers, thereby eliminating the division between public and private insurance for basic population cover.

Private health insurance offers 88% of the French population *complementary* insurance to cover cost-sharing in the social security system. The Netherlands has the largest *supplementary* market (92% of the population), followed by Canada (67%) whereby private insurance pays for prescription drugs and dental care that are not publicly reimbursed. Approximately one-third of the Austrian and Swiss populations also have supplementary health insurance. *Duplicate* markets providing faster private-sector access to medical services where there are waiting times in public systems are largest in Ireland (51%), Australia (44%) and New Zealand (33%). The population covered by private health insurance is positively correlated to the share of total health spending accounted for by private health insurance (Figure 6.2.3).

The importance of private health insurance is not linked to a countries' economic development. Other factors are more likely to explain market development, including gaps in access to publicly financed services, the way private providers are financed, government interventions directed at private health insurance markets, and historical development (OECD, 2004b).

Definition and deviations

Population coverage is the share of the population receiving a defined set of health care goods and services under public programmes and private health insurance. It includes those covered in their own name and their dependents. Public coverage refers both to government programmes, generally financed by taxation, and social health insurance, generally financed by payroll taxes. Take-up of private health insurance is often voluntary, although it may be mandatory by law or compulsory for employees as part of their working conditions. Premiums are generally non-income-related, although the purchase of private cover can be subsidised by the government.

6.2.1 Health insurance coverage for a core set of services, 2007

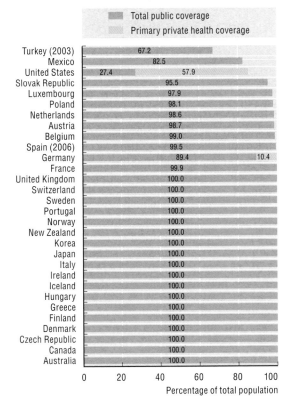

Total public coverage
Primary private health coverage

6.2.2 Private health insurance coverage, by type, 2007

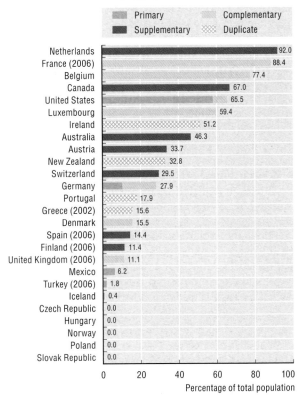

Primary   Complementary
Supplementary   Duplicate

Note: Private health insurance can be both duplicate and supplementary in Australia; and can be both complementary and supplementary in Denmark.

Source: OECD Health Data 2009, OECD Survey of Health System Characteristics 2008-2009.

6.2.3 Private health insurance, population covered and share in total health expenditure, 2007

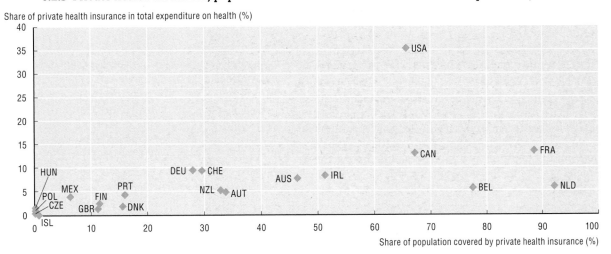

Source: OECD Health Data 2009.

StatLink ᘓᓫ᠊ http://dx.doi.org/10.1787/720176631305

Financial protection through public or private health insurance substantially reduces the amount that people pay directly for medical care, yet in some countries the burden of out-of-pocket spending can still create barriers to health care access and use. Households that have difficulties paying medical bills may delay or forgo needed health care (Hoffman *et al.*, 2005; May and Cunningham, in Banthin *et al.*, 2008). On average across OECD countries, 18% of health spending is paid directly by patients (see Indicator 7.6 "Financing of health care").

In contrast to publicly-funded care, out-of-pocket payments rely on the ability to pay. If the financing of health care becomes more dependent on out-of-pocket payments, its burden is, in theory, shifted towards those who use services more, possibly from high to low income earners, where health care needs are higher. In practice, many countries have exemptions and caps to out-of-pocket payments for lower income groups to protect health care access. Switzerland, for example, has a high proportion of out-of-pocket expenditure, but it has cost-sharing exemptions for large families, social-assistance beneficiaries and others. There is an annual cap on deductibles and co-insurance payments (OECD and WHO, 2006).

The burden of out-of-pocket health spending can be measured either by its share of total household income or its share of total household consumption. The average share varied considerably across OECD countries in 2007, representing less than 2% of total household consumption in countries such as the Netherlands and France, but almost 6% in Switzerland and Greece (Figure 6.3.1). The United States, with almost 3% of consumption being spent on out-of-pocket health services, is close to the average. In 2007, 30% of US adults paid more than USD 1 000 in out-of-pocket medical costs over the past year, while only 4% of UK adults paid similar amounts (Figure 6.3.2). In some central and eastern European countries, the practice of unofficial supplementary payments means that the level of out-of-pocket spending may be underestimated.

The distribution of spending across the population can vary markedly, although data is only available for a small number of countries. The US Medical Expenditure Panel Survey found that 28% of Americans living in a poor family (defined as a family income below the Federal poverty level) were spending more than 10% of their after-tax family income for health services and health insurance premiums in 2004, compared with 10% of Americans in a high income family (Banthin *et al.*, 2008). Similarly, 5% of Belgian households in the lowest

income decile spent more than 10% of their gross income on out-of-pocket payments in 1997, compared to less than 1% of households in the highest decile (De Graeve and Van Ourti, 2003). In 2004, households in the lowest income quartile in the Netherlands spent 3.4% of their disposable income on out-of-pocket payments; in the highest quartile this was 2% (Westert *et al.*, 2008).

A small proportion of households in OECD countries face "catastrophic" health expenditure each year, perhaps as a result of severe illness or major injury. Catastrophic health expenditure is commonly defined as payments for health services exceeding 40% of household disposable income after subsistence needs are met (Xu *et al.*, 2007). Countries that have a greater reliance on out-of-pocket health care expenditure tend also to have a higher proportion of households with catastrophic expenditure (Figure 6.3.3). In Portugal, Spain, Switzerland and the United States, rates of catastrophic spending exceed five per 1 000 people (Xu *et al.*, 2007). In Mexico, the high level of out-of-pocket spending resulted in 3.4% of households having catastrophic health expenditure in 2003; among the lowest income quintile this rose to 4.7%, and among uninsured persons it was 5.1% (OECD, 2005c). In some countries, the imposition of user fees may mean that lower income households forgo health care altogether, and thus not use enough services to incur catastrophic expenditures.

Definition and deviations

Out-of-pocket payments are expenditures borne directly by a patient where insurance does not cover the full cost of the health good or service. They include cost-sharing, self-medication and other expenditure paid directly by private households. In some countries they also include estimations of informal payments to health care providers. Some households face very high out-of-pocket payments. Catastrophic health expenditure is commonly defined as payments for health services exceeding 40% of household disposable income after subsistence needs are met.

Information on of out-of-pocket expenditure is collected through household expenditure surveys in a number of OECD countries.

6.3.1 Out-of-pocket expenditure as a share of final household consumption, 2007 (or nearest available year)

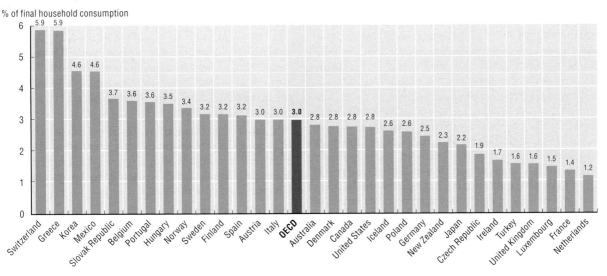

% of final household consumption

Source: OECD Health Data 2009.

6.3.2 Out-of-pocket medical costs in the past year, seven OECD countries, 2007

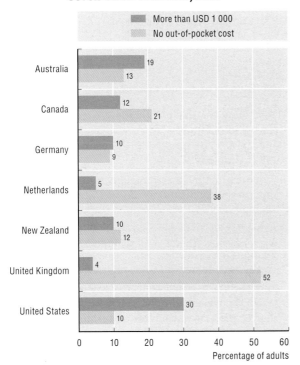

Source: 2007 Commonwealth Fund International Health Policy Survey.

6.3.3 Catastrophic expenditure and out-of-pocket payments for health care, late 1990s

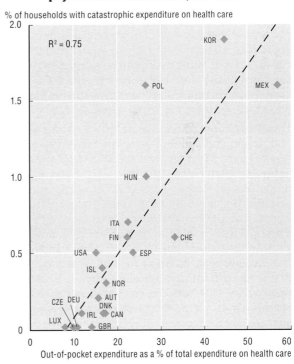

% of households with catastrophic expenditure on health care

Source: Xu et al. (2007); OECD Health Data 2009.

StatLink ᤰ᠊ᡗᡅ http://dx.doi.org/10.1787/720205046358

Access to medical care requires an adequate number and proper distribution of physicians across the country. Shortages of physicians in a geographic region can lead to increased travel times for patients and higher caseloads for doctors, which may result in increased waiting times to receive care. Measuring disparities in the "density" of physicians among regions within the same country gives some indication of the accessibility of doctor services. Regions, however, may contain a mixture of urban and rural populations, so that although a region may have high physician density, persons living in geographically remote areas of that region may still face long travel times to receive medical care. In addition, the services that physicians offer should match need, whether these are for GPs or specialists.

OECD countries display very different levels in the number of practising physicians per 1 000 population, ranging from lows of less than two in Turkey, Korea and Mexico, to highs of four and more in Belgium and Greece (see Figure 3.2.1 for Indicator 3.2 "Practising physicians").

In many countries, there is a greater number of physicians per capita in the national capital than in other regions (Figure 6.4.1). In the Czech Republic for example, Prague has a density of physicians almost twice the country average. The regional distribution of physicians is fairly even in Japan and Poland (OECD, 2009e). There is also disparity in the density of specialists, with a greater concentration evident in capital cities in a number of countries, such as Mexico, the Slovak Republic and Turkey (Figure 6.4.2).

The density of physicians is greater in regions with a high urban population, due to the concentration of services such as surgery and specialised practitioners in metropolitan centres (Figure 6.4.3). In Canada, just under 16% of "family physicians" (mostly general practitioners) and only 2% of specialists were located in rural areas and small towns in 2006, whereas 24% of the population resided in these areas (Dumont et al., 2008). In the United States, 17% of the population lived in non-metropolitan areas in 2004, but only 9% of practising patient care physicians were located in these areas. There also tends to be fewer specialists outside cities – almost 50% of US counties had no obstetricians or gynaecologists providing direct patient care in 2004 (NCHS, 2007). The situation is similar in France, with 22% of general practitioners and 4% of specialists practising in towns of up to 10 000 population in 2007, whereas 36% of the population resided in these areas (DREES, 2008).

In Australia, primary care physicians (mostly general practitioners) are fairly evenly distributed, ranging from an estimated 100 full-time equivalent per 100 000 population in major cities in 2005, to 88 in inner regional, 84 in outer regional and 92 in remote/very remote regions. Specialists, however, ranged from 122 in major cities, to 56 in inner regional, 38 in outer regional and only 16 in remote/very remote regions (AIHW, 2008c).

A number of factors are likely to affect the distribution of physicians. These include the population size and economic development of a region, the regions' professional climate and the extent of social amenities in a region (Huber et al., 2008).

Experience shows that a mix of policies are needed to address maldistribution issues (Simoens and Hurst, 2006). In Canada, for example, foreign-trained doctors comprised an average of 30% of the labour force in rural and remote areas in 2006. Incentives have also been developed to train health professionals with rural background and exposure (Dumont et al., 2008). In Turkey, significant numbers of new health staff have been assigned to areas with low physician density in recent years, although the challenge remains to match staff with areas of greatest need (OECD and the World Bank, 2008).

Definition and deviations

Practising physicians include general practitioners and specialists who are actively practising medicine. For more detail, see Indicator 3.2 "Practising physicians".

Since countries use a variety of different geographical classifications, the OECD has classified regions within each member country into two territorial levels. The higher level (Territorial Level 2) consists of 335 large regions within the 30 member countries. For the most part, these correspond to national administrative regions.

Further sub-regional analysis may be necessary to obtain a more complete picture of geographic distribution of physicians. A number of countries have developed schemes to classify populations into urban-rural categories, although these are not standard, making cross-national comparisons difficult.

6.4.1 Physician density, by Territorial Level 2 regions, 2005

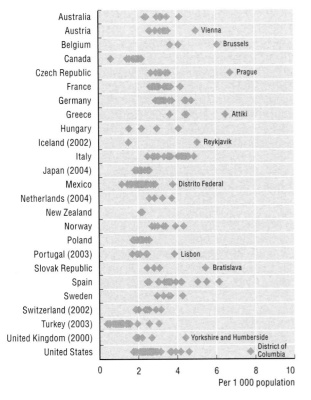

Source: OECD Regions at a Glance 2009.

6.4.2 Specialist density, by Territorial Level 2 regions, selected OECD countries, 2004

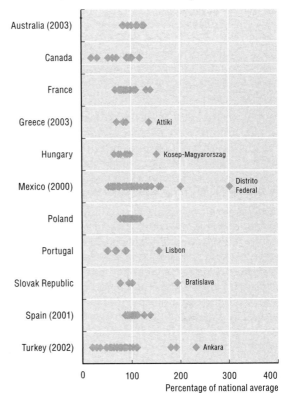

Source: OECD Regions at a Glance 2009.

6.4.3 Physician density in rural and urban regions, four OECD countries, 2005 (or nearest year)

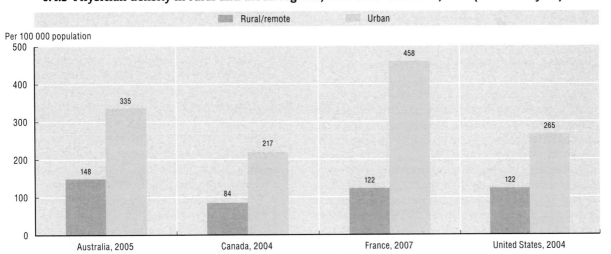

Note: Classifications of rural and urban regions differ between countries.
Source: AIHW (2008c); CIHI (2005); DREES (2008); NCHS (2007).

StatLink http://dx.doi.org/10.1787/720216814125

Measuring rates of health care utilisation, such as doctor consultations, is one way of identifying whether there are access problems for certain populations. Difficulties in consulting doctors because of excess cost, long waiting periods or travelling time, lack of knowledge or incentive may lead to lower utilisation, and in turn to poorer health status and increased health inequalities.

The average number of consultations per capita varies greatly across OECD countries (see Indicator 4.1 "Consultations with doctors"). But there are also significant differences among population groups within countries. One dimension that is often used to examine these variations is socio-economic status, as determined by income, education, or occupation.

A study by van Doorslaer et al. (2004) examined income-related inequality in visits to doctors in a number of OECD countries around the year 2000. After adjusting for differences in need for health care (since health problems are more frequent and more severe among people from lower socio-economic groups), doctor visits were found to be more frequent among higher income persons in nine out of 21 countries – Canada, Finland, Italy, Mexico, the Netherlands, Norway, Portugal, Sweden and the United States – but the degree of inequity was fairly small. In the other 12 OECD countries, given the same need, high income people were as likely to see a doctor as those with low income. A similar study using 1998 data found income-related equity for doctor visits in Korea (Lu et al., 2007).

For a majority of countries in the study, data were available for both GP and specialist visits. GP visits were equitably distributed in most countries, and when significant inequity existed it was often negative, favouring low income earners (Figure 6.5.1). However, a different story emerged for specialist visits – in nearly all countries, high income people were more likely to see a specialist than those with low income (Figure 6.5.2), and in most countries also more frequently (van Doorslaer et al., 2004; 2008). In Europe, this was especially so in Portugal, Finland, Ireland and Italy, four countries where private insurance and direct private payments played an important role in accessing specialist services. In Finland, the sources of these socio-economic differences in specialist visits include the size of patient co-payments, the pro-high income distribution of workplace services that facilitate access to specialist care, and the large private ambulatory care sector (NOMESCO, 2004; OECD, 2005b).

Consistent with these findings, research in 13 European countries has found that, after control-

ling for need, people with higher education levels tend to use specialist care more, and the same was true for GP use in several countries (including France, Portugal and Hungary) (Or et al., 2008). The study suggests that, beyond the direct cost of care, other health system characteristics are important in reducing social inequities in health care utilisation, such as the role given to the GP and the organisation of primary care. Social inequalities in specialist use were found to be less in countries with a National Health System and where GPs act as gatekeepers. Countries with established primary care networks may place greater emphasis on meeting the care needs of deprived populations, and gatekeeping often provides simpler access and better guidance for people in lower socio-economic positions (Or et al., 2008).

A more recent study from Canada for 2003 confirmed that higher income persons had inequitably higher rates of GP and specialist consultations (Allin, 2006). On the other hand, no significant differences in the use of GP or specialist care was found between people with higher and lower education levels in the Netherlands in 2005 (Westert et al., 2008).

Definition and deviations

Consultations with doctors refer to the number of ambulatory contacts with physicians (both generalists and specialists). For more information, see Indicator 4.1 "Consultations with doctors".

Estimates in studies by van Doorslaer et al. (2004) and Or et al. (2008) come from health interview or household surveys conducted around 2000, and rely on self-report. Inequalities in doctor consultations are assessed in terms of people's income and educational level. The number of doctor consultations is adjusted for need, based on self-reported information about health status.

Differing survey questions and response categories may affect the ability to make valid cross-national comparisons. Surveyed groups may vary in age range, and the measures used to grade income and education level can also vary. Caution is therefore needed when interpreting inequalities in health care utilisation across countries.

6.5.1 Horizontal inequity indices for probability of a GP visit (with 95% confidence interval), 17 OECD countries, 2000 (or nearest available year)

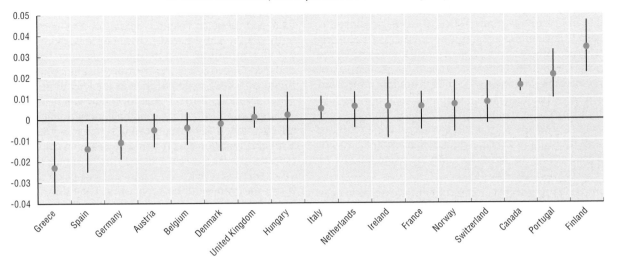

6.5.2 Horizontal inequity indices for probability of a specialist visit (with 95% confidence interval), 17 OECD countries, 2000 (or nearest available year)

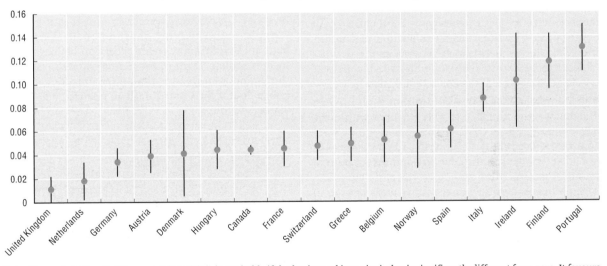

Note: The probability of a GP or specialist visit is inequitable if the horizontal inequity index is significantly different from zero. It favours low income groups when it is below zero, and high income groups when it is above zero. The index is adjusted for need.

Source: Van Doorslaer *et al.* (2004).

StatLink ⬛ *http://dx.doi.org/10.1787/720237010637*

Dental caries, periodontal (gum) disease and tooth loss are common problems in OECD countries, variously affecting almost all adults and 60-90% of school children (see Indicator 1.10 "Dental health among children"). Despite great improvements problems persist, occurring most commonly among disadvantaged and low income groups. In the United States for example, almost 50% of low income persons aged 20-64 years had untreated dental caries in 2001-04, compared with only 20% of high income persons (NCHS, 2009). In Finland, one-quarter of adults with lower education were found to have six or more missing teeth, while less than 10% of those with higher education had the same amount of tooth loss (Kaikkonen, 2007).

Strategies to improve access to dental care for disadvantaged or underserviced populations include reducing financial and non-financial barriers, and promoting an adequate dental workforce in all regions to respond to demand.

In most OECD countries, public health authorities recommend an annual visit to a dentist. The average number of per capita consultations with dentists varied widely in 2007, from over three in Japan and over two in Belgium, to 0.2 in Turkey (2002) and 0.1 in Mexico, with an OECD average of 1.3 (Figure 6.6.1). Some of this variation can be explained by the differing availability of dentists. In general, as the number of dentists increases, so does the number of consultations per capita (see Indicator 3.11 "Dentists").

Van Doorslaer et al. (2004) found that high income persons were more likely to visit a dentist within the last 12 months, in all OECD countries where data were available (Figure 6.6.2). This was despite differences in public and private dental coverage and the amount of reimbursement. There was, however, wide variation. At the time of this study, inequalities were smaller in countries with a higher probability of a dental visit such as Sweden and the Netherlands, and larger in Portugal, the United States, Finland and Canada.

Sweden was the most equitable country for the probability of a dental visit. Dental care is largely subsidised through a national dental insurance system. Free care is provided for children and young people to age 19, and a number of services, including prosthetic treatment, are fully subsidised for older people. Reforms in July 2008 have extended care by introducing vouchers for people aged 20 years and over, as well as a high-cost protection scheme. In 2006, Sweden spent 3.4% of public expenditure on health on dental services, well ahead of the OECD average of 2.5%.

In the United States, more recent data confirms the wide differences between income groups in the probability of a dental visit. Less than half of poor and near-poor persons visited a dentist in 2006 compared with 70% of middle and high income persons. This gap has remained largely unchanged over the past decade (Figure 6.6.3). As in many other countries, financial access to dental care in the United States is generally more difficult than for medical care, since a smaller proportion of persons have dental insurance. In 2001, only 61% of American adults had some form of dental insurance, compared to 86% of adults with medical insurance. On average in 2003, one-half of total dental care costs were paid out-of-pocket (NCHS, 2007), and more adults report that they did not get needed dental care due to costs than medical care (see Indicator 6.1 "Unmet health care needs").

Oral health care is mostly provided by private dental practitioners. Treatment is costly, averaging 6% of total health expenditure (and 16% of private health expenditure) across OECD countries in 2006. In countries such as Australia, Canada and New Zealand, adult dental care is not part of the basic packages of services which is included in public care insurance. In other countries, prevention and treatment are covered, but a varying share of costs is born by patients, and this may create access problems for low-income groups (Figure 6.6.4). Some countries, such as the Nordic countries and the United Kingdom, provide public dental care, particularly to children and disadvantaged groups.

Definition and deviations

Consultations with dentists refer to the probability and the number of contacts with dentists. Estimates usually come from health interview or household surveys, and rely on self-report, although some countries provide administrative data. Inequalities in dental consultations are here assessed in terms of people's income.

Differing survey questions and response categories may affect the ability to make valid cross-national comparisons. Surveyed groups may vary in age range, and the measures used to grade income level can also vary. Caution is therefore needed when interpreting inequalities across countries.

6.6.1 Average number of dentist consultations per capita, 2007 (or latest year available)

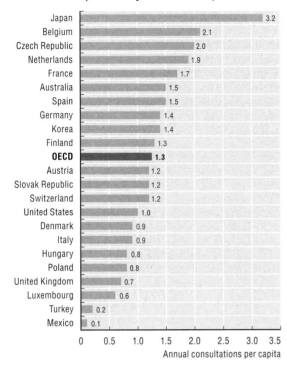

Annual consultations per capita

Source: OECD Health Data 2009.

6.6.2 Probability of a dental visit in the past 12 months, by income group, 18 OECD countries, 2000 (or latest year available)

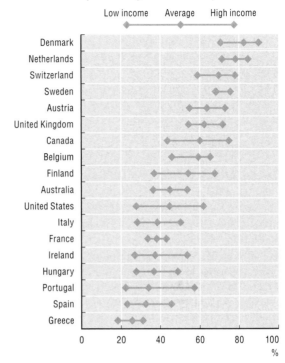

Source: Van Doorslaer et al. (2004).

6.6.3 Proportion of adults visiting a dentist in the past year, by income group, United States, 1997-2006

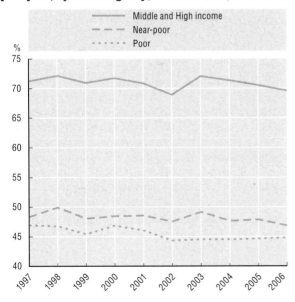

Source: NCHS (2009).

6.6.4 Out-of-pocket dental expenditure, 2006 (or latest year available)

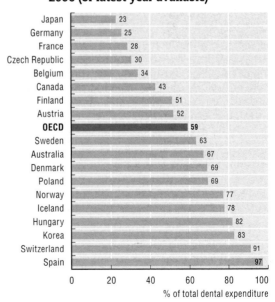

% of total dental expenditure

Source: OECD Health Data 2009.

StatLink ⌨ http://dx.doi.org/10.1787/720242166871

Cancer is the second most common cause of death in OECD countries, responsible for 27% of all deaths in 2006. Among women, breast cancer is the most common form, accounting for 30% or more of new cases each year and 16% of cancer deaths in 2006. Cervical cancer accounts for an additional 5% of new cases, and 3% of female cancer deaths (see Indicator 1.5 "Mortality from Cancer").

The early detection of breast and cervical cancers through screening programmes has contributed significantly to increased survival rates and declines in mortality from these diseases, and many countries have opted to make screening widely available. In most countries, more than half of women in the target age groups for screening have had a recent mammogram, and pelvic exam or Pap smear (see Indicator 5.7 "Screening, survival and mortality for cervical cancer" and Indicator 5.8 "Screening, survival and mortality for breast cancer").

Screening rates vary widely among women in different socio-economic groups in OECD countries (Figures 6.7.1 and 6.7.2). In the United States, low income women, women who are uninsured or receiving Medicaid (health insurance coverage for the poor, disabled or impoverished elderly) or women with lower educational levels report much lower use of mammography and Pap smears (NCHS, 2009). Even in those countries where the practice is common, women in the lowest wealth quintiles are generally less likely to undergo screening (Gakidou et al., 2008; WHO, 2008b). There are exceptions, with women in the lowest wealth quintiles in Luxembourg and the Netherlands as likely to have had a mammogram as those in higher wealth quintiles. The same is true regarding cervical cancer screening in the Czech Republic, Italy and the United Kingdom.

Participation rates also vary by geographic regions (Figure 6.7.3). Some areas, such as the Northern Territory (Australia), and London (United Kingdom), exhibit significantly lower rates than do other regions within the country (AIHW, 2008a; NHSBSP, 2008). The reasons for this are varied. In geographically isolated regions, travelling distance and number of available screening facilities play a part. In inner urban areas, low levels of awareness of screening programmes, symptoms and risks are a concern among women who are poor, or from minority ethnic groups.

A number of socio-economic characteristics – such as income, ethnicity, younger age, higher level of education, employment status, residential area, marital status, having health insurance, good health status, having a usual source of care and use of other preventative services – are all important predictors of participation in screening.

In Mexico, cervical cancer detection programmes have been in place for some time, but problems with access and coverage remain, especially among disadvantaged groups, so that almost half of women aged 50 years and over have not had a Pap test in the last two years (Couture et al., 2008). In most OECD countries, however, income should not be a barrier to accessing screening mammography or Pap smears, since the services are provided free of charge, or at the cost of a doctor consultation.

Since a wide range of screening practices and different access barriers exist across OECD countries, no single strategy will meet all needs in promoting greater and equal coverage (Gakidou et al., 2008). In countries with sufficient health system capacity, increased screening can be encouraged by ensuring services are free, and are available where needed. Policies and interventions may need to be better targeted in order to overcome inequalities. As a complementary tool, the promise of new cancer preventing vaccines also has important implications for resource-poor settings where maintaining screening programmes is challenging.

Definition and deviations

Breast and cervical screening participation rates measure the proportion of women of a given age who have variously received a recent mammogram, breast exam, Pap smear or pelvic exam. Information is generally derived from health surveys, or from screening programme administrative data.

For this indicator, rates by wealth quintiles were derived from health surveys of women aged 25-64 years (cervical) and 50-69 years (breast) who reported that they had been screened in the three years prior to the survey. Screening estimates based on self-reported health surveys should be used cautiously, since respondents tend to overestimate desirable behaviours.

The data for geographic regions include women in target age groups who had participated in national screening programmes. Target age groups and screening periodicity may differ across countries.

6.7.1 Cervical cancer screening in selected OECD countries, by wealth quintile, 2002-04

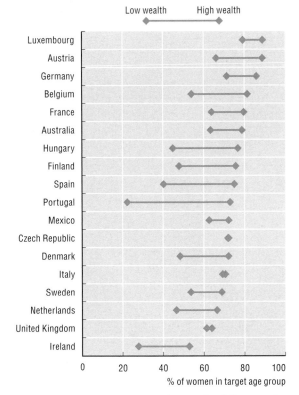

6.7.2 Breast cancer screening in selected OECD countries, by wealth quintile, 2002-04

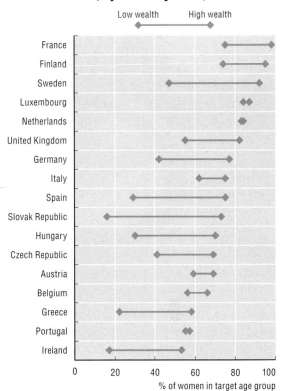

Note: The data source for some countries may be different to that used for reporting breast and cervical cancer screening in Chapter 5. Since these studies were conducted, a number of countries, including Ireland, have introduced national population-based screening.

Source: Gakidou *et al.* (2008).

Source: WHO (2008b).

6.7.3 Participation in breast cancer screening programmes, regions in selected OECD countries

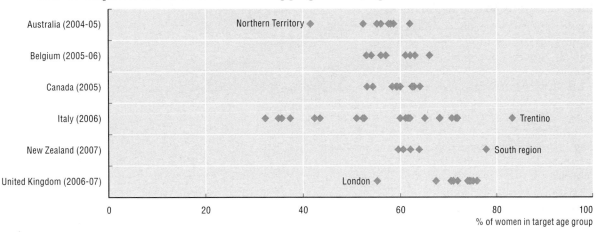

Source: AIHW (2008a); IMA-AIM (2009); PHAC (2008); ONS (2008); Taylor *et al.* (2008); NHSBSP (2008).

StatLink *http://dx.doi.org/10.1787/720281253448*

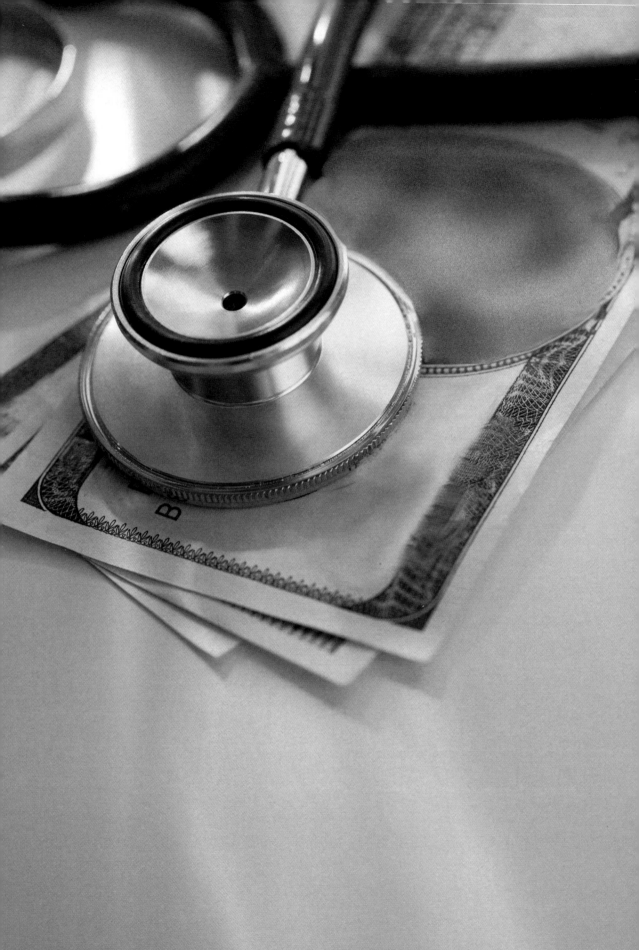

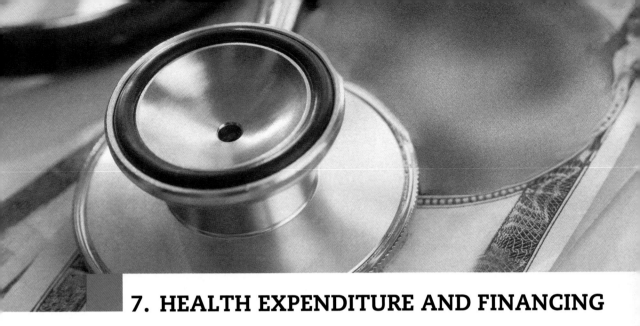

7. HEALTH EXPENDITURE AND FINANCING

Introduction

This chapter presents an overview of the main indicators and characteristics of health spending and financing across OECD countries.

The discussion starts with a comparison of overall health spending in terms of per capita expenditure and in relation to other macroeconomic variables, such as GDP. Current levels of spending as well as trends over recent years are presented, taking into account the likely impact of the economic slowdown on future health spending. As well as indicators of total spending, the chapter also provides an analysis of the different types of health services and goods consumed across OECD countries, with a separate focus on pharmaceuticals as one of the main drivers of health spending growth over recent years.

A new and important area included in this version of *Health at a Glance* is health care expenditure broken down according to patients' characteristics, or more particularly, disease conditions and age. Such analysis is key for health policy makers in order to show current resource allocation in the health care system. The information provided can play an important role in discussions concerning changing demographics and disease patterns, as well as the modelling of future health care expenditures. Along with the allocation of health care spending, the chapter also addresses the question of "where does the money come from?", *i.e.* where the burden for paying for such goods and services lies. Finally, with the growth in medical tourism and international trade in health services, current levels and trends are examined in the light of efforts to improve data availability and coverage to feed growing policy needs.

Comparison of health expenditure and financing across countries

The vast majority of countries now produce health spending data according to the boundaries and definitions proposed in the OECD manual *A System of Health Accounts* (OECD, 2000). The comparability of the functional breakdown of health expenditure data has improved over recent years. However, limitations remain, as some countries have not yet implemented the SHA classifications and definitions. Even among those countries that are submitting data according to the SHA, the comparability of data may be less than optimal. For example, in-patient expenditure does not contain independent billing of physicians' fees for in-patient care in Canada and the United States. Different practices regarding the inclusion of long-term care in health or social expenditure are also a factor affecting data comparability.

Regarding the functional breakdown of health expenditure presented in this publication, out-patient expenditure is used in a broad sense to cover both out-patient care in a hospital setting as well as in the ambulatory sector.

For further information, see the "Note on General Comparability of Health Expenditure and Finance Data" in *OECD Health Data 2009*.

Definition of health expenditure

Total expenditure on health measures the final consumption of health care goods and services plus capital investment in health care infrastructure. This includes spending by both public and private sources (including households) on medical services and goods, public health and prevention programmes and administration.

The following table lists the major expenditure categories according to the International Classification for Health Accounts (ICHA) used in *OECD Health Data 2009* and presented in this publication.

ICHA code	Description
HC.1; HC.2	Services of curative and rehabilitative care (in-patient, day care, out-patient and home care)
HC.3	Services of long-term nursing care (in-patient, day care and home care)
HC.4	Ancillary services to health care
HC.1-HC.4	Medical services
HC.5	Medical goods dispensed to outpatients
HC.1-HC.5	Total expenditure on personal health
HC.6	Services of prevention and public health
HC.7	Health administration and health insurance
HC.6 + HC.7	Total expenditure on collective health
HC.1-HC.7	Total current expenditure on health
HC.R.1	Capital formation (Investment) in health care provider institutions
HC.1-HC.7 + HC.R.1	TOTAL EXPENDITURE ON HEALTH

Adjustment for differences in national currency

Health expenditure based on national currency units can be used for comparing some indicators, such as the ratio of health expenditure to GDP and health spending growth rates over time.

However, to make useful comparisons of health expenditure across countries at a given point in time, it is necessary to convert data from national currency units to a common currency, such as the US dollar (USD). It is also useful to take into account differences in the purchasing power of national currencies in each country. To calculate the conversion rate of national currencies into US dollar purchasing power parity (PPP), the same, fixed basket of goods and services across different countries is priced in the national currency, and then converted to US dollars. For example, if an identical basket of goods and services cost 140 Canadian dollars (CAD) in Canada and USD 100 in the United States, then the PPP conversion rate would be CAD 1.4 to USD 1. The economy-wide (GDP) PPPs are used as the most available and reliable conversion rates. These are based on a broad basket of goods and services, chosen to be representative of all economic activity. The use of economy-wide PPPs means that the resulting variations in health expenditure across countries will reflect not only variations in the volume of health services, but also any variations in the prices of health services relative to prices in the rest of the economy.

With regard to imports and exports of health goods and services, data are expressed in US dollars converted at market exchange rates.

Correcting data for price inflation

To make useful comparisons of real growth rates over time, it is necessary to deflate (*i.e.* remove inflation from) nominal health expenditure through the use of a suitable price index, and also to divide by the population, to derive real spending per capita. Due to the limited availability of reliable health price indices, an economy-wide (GDP) price index is used in this publication, at 2000 GDP price levels.

7.1. Health expenditure per capita

Differences in spending levels per capita reflect a wide array of market and social factors, as well as countries' diverse financing and organisational structures of their health systems.

The United States continues to outspend all other OECD countries by a wide margin. In 2007, spending on health goods and services per person in the United States rose to USD 7 290 (Figure 7.1.1) – almost two and a half times the average of all OECD countries. Norway and Switzerland spend about two-thirds of the per capita level of the United States, but are still around 50% above the OECD average. Most of the northern and western European countries, together with Canada and Australia, spend between USD PPP 3 000 and 4 000, between 100% and 130% of the OECD average. Those countries spending below the OECD average include Mexico and Turkey, but also the southern and eastern European members of the OECD together with Korea. Japan also spends less on health than the average in OECD countries, despite its above-average per capita income.

Figure 7.1.1 also shows the breakdown of per capita spending on health into public and private components (see also Indicator 7.6). The variation in the levels of public spending on health is similar to that observed for total spending on health. In general, the ranking according to per capita public expenditure remains comparable to that of total spending. Even if the private sector in the United States continues to play the dominant role in financing, public spending on health per capita is still greater than that in most other OECD countries (with the exception of Norway and Luxembourg), because overall spending on health is much higher than in other countries.

In Switzerland, a large proportion of health care financing comes from private sources, and its public spending on health as a share of GDP is lower than in certain other countries, although overall spending is higher. The opposite is true in Denmark where most health care is publically financed.

Per capita health spending over 1997-2007 is estimated to have grown, in real terms, by 4.1% annually on average across the OECD (Figure 7.1.2, Table A.10). In many countries, the growth rate reached a peak around 2001-02 and slowed in more recent years. By comparison, average economic growth over this period was 2.6%, resulting in an increasing share of the economy devoted to health in most countries (Figure 7.1.3; see also Indicator 7.2).

In general, the countries that have experienced the highest growth in health expenditures per capita over this period are those that had relatively low levels at the beginning of the period. Health expenditure growth in Korea and Turkey, for example, has been more than twice the OECD average over the past ten years. Other countries, such as Ireland and the United Kingdom, pursued specific policy objectives to increase public spending on health, meaning that overall health spending has outpaced economic growth (Department of Health and Children, 2001; Secretary of State for Health, 2002).

In Germany, health spending per capita increased, in real terms, by only 1.7% per year on average, reflecting the effect of cost-containment policies designed to achieve stable contribution rates by employers and employees. These measures have included budget or spending caps for sectors or individual providers, introducing reference prices for pharmaceuticals and educational approaches to enhance generic and rational prescribing, reducing the number of hospital beds and restricting the number of high cost medical equipment, and introducing or increasing co-payments for certain services (Busse and Riesberg, 2004).

Definition and deviations

Total expenditure on health measures the final consumption of health goods and services (i.e. current health expenditure) plus capital investment in health care infrastructure. This includes spending by both public and private sources on medical services and goods, public health and prevention programmes and administration.

Countries' health expenditures are converted to a common currency (US dollar) and adjusted to take account of the different purchasing power of the national currencies, in order to compare spending levels. Economy-wide (GDP) PPPs are used as the most available and reliable conversion rates.

The growth rates presented in Figures 7.1.2 and 7.1.3 have been adjusted to take account of series breaks that are in most cases due to the implementation of the *System of Health Accounts*. To remove these breaks, the real growth in the year of the series break has been assumed to be the average growth of the preceding and following years.

7.1.1 Total health expenditure per capita, public and private, 2007

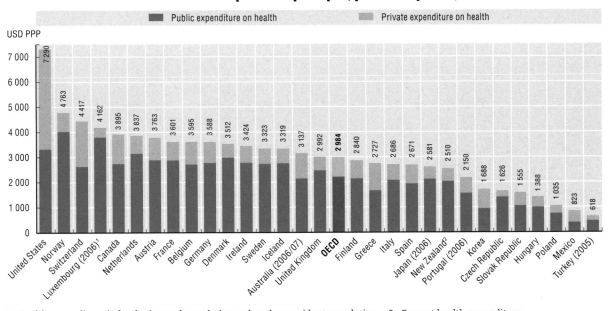

1. Health expenditure is for the insured population rather than resident population.   2. Current health expenditure.

7.1.2 Annual average real growth in per capita health expenditure, 1997-2007

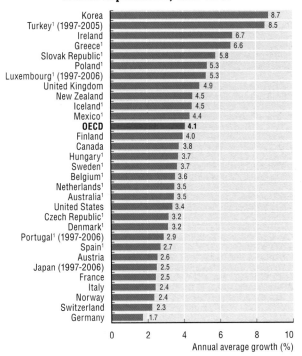

1. Growth rates adjusted. See box "Definition and deviations".

7.1.3 Annual average real growth in per capita health expenditure and GDP, 1997-2007

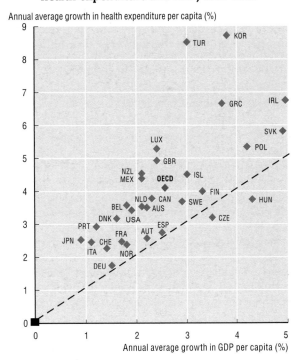

Source: OECD Health Data 2009.

StatLink ⟦⟧ http://dx.doi.org/10.1787/720324283737

In 2007, OECD countries devoted 8.9% of their GDP to health spending (Figure 7.2.1). Trends in the health spending to GDP ratio are the result of the combined effect of trends in both GDP and health expenditure. Apart from a few countries (Hungary and the Czech Republic), health spending grew more quickly than GDP over the last ten years (see Figure 7.1.3 under the previous indicator). This has resulted in a higher share of GDP allocated to health (Figure 7.2.3). The share of health expenditure to GDP is likely to increase further, following the recession that started in many countries in 2008 and became widespread in 2009.

In 2007, the share of health spending to GDP ranged from less than 6% in Turkey and Mexico up to 16% of GDP in the United States (Figure 7.2.1 and Table A.12). Following the United States were France (11.0%), Switzerland (10.8%), and Germany (10.4%).

The share of public expenditure on health to GDP also varies from a high of 8.7% of GDP in France to lows of 3.7% and 2.7% of GDP in Korea and Mexico, respectively. In these two countries, health spending is almost evenly split between public and private financing.

To make a more comprehensive assessment of health spending, the health spending to GDP ratio should be considered together with per capita health spending (see Indicator 7.1 "Health expenditure per capita"). Countries having a relatively high health spending to GDP ratio might have relatively low health expenditure per capita, and the converse also holds. For example, Austria and Portugal both spent approximately 10% of their GDP on health; however, per capita spending (adjusted to USD PPP) was almost 70% higher in Austria (Figure 7.1.1).

Figure 7.2.4 shows a positive association between GDP per capita and health expenditure per capita across OECD countries. While there is an overall tendency for countries with higher GDP to spend a greater amount on health, there is wide variation since GDP is not the sole factor influencing health expenditure levels. The association is stronger among OECD countries with low GDP per capita than among countries with a higher GDP per capita. Even for countries with similar levels of GDP per capita there are substantial differences in health expenditure at a given level of GDP. For example, despite Japan and Germany having similar GDP per capita, their health spending per capita differs considerably with Japan spending less than 75% of the level of Germany on health.

The reduction in GDP, due to the economic downturn, may lead to rises in the health spending to GDP ratios in the short term. There is little evidence that GDP changes have an impact on the *level* of health spending in the short term. However, the experience of some OECD countries that have faced substantial recessions in the past 20 years is that health expenditures may be reduced in the following years.

The health spending to GDP ratio does not accurately measure the relative magnitude of health goods and services consumed by individuals because, firstly, total health expenditure includes investments made by health providers, and secondly, GDP includes also net exports. A more refined measure of the relative importance of health spending is the share of health goods and services to all the goods and services consumed by individuals in the economy, regardless of who paid for them. This ratio is notably higher than the total health expenditure to GDP ratio for all OECD countries (Figure 7.2.2). The average share of actual consumption allocated to health across OECD countries is almost 13%, with the vast majority of OECD countries devoting more than 10% of their consumption to health. Five countries (United States, Switzerland, Luxembourg, Norway and Austria) spent more than 15% on health in 2007.

Definition and deviations

Gross Domestic Product (GDP) = final consumption + gross capital formation + net exports. Actual final consumption of households includes goods and services used by households or the community to satisfy their individual needs. It includes final consumption expenditure of households, general government and non-profit institutions serving households.

Differences in the relative positions of countries according to the ratio of total health expenditure to GDP and current health expenditure to actual final consumption expenditure are due to differences in the level of investments (in the economy as a whole, and in the health sector), in the balance of foreign trade across countries, and in net income from abroad. These adjustments are significant for countries such as Luxembourg, Ireland and Norway.

7.2.1 Total health expenditure as a share of GDP, 2007

7.2.2 Current health expenditure as a share of household consumption, 2007

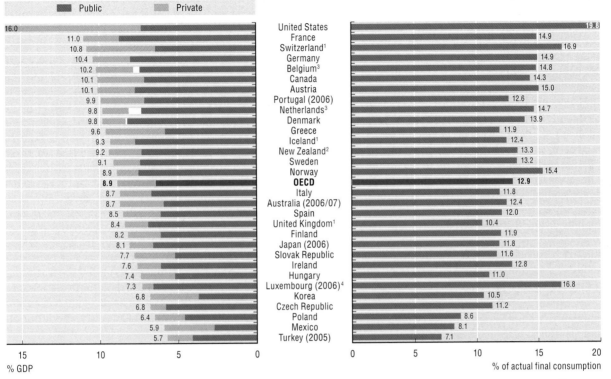

	% GDP		% of actual final consumption
United States	16.0		19.8
France	11.0		14.9
Switzerland[1]	10.8		16.9
Germany	10.4		14.9
Belgium[3]	10.2		14.8
Canada	10.1		14.3
Austria	10.1		15.0
Portugal (2006)	9.9		12.6
Netherlands[3]	9.8		14.7
Denmark	9.8		13.9
Greece	9.6		11.9
Iceland[1]	9.3		12.4
New Zealand[2]	9.2		13.3
Sweden	9.1		13.2
Norway	8.9		15.4
OECD	**8.9**		**12.9**
Italy	8.7		11.8
Australia (2006/07)	8.7		12.4
Spain	8.5		12.0
United Kingdom[1]	8.4		10.4
Finland	8.2		11.9
Japan (2006)	8.1		11.8
Slovak Republic	7.7		11.6
Ireland	7.6		12.8
Hungary	7.4		11.0
Luxembourg (2006)[4]	7.3		16.8
Korea	6.8		10.5
Czech Republic	6.8		11.2
Poland	6.4		8.6
Mexico	5.9		8.1
Turkey (2005)	5.7		7.1

1. Total expenditure on health in both figures.   2. Current expenditure on health in both figures.   3. Public and private expenditures are current expenditures (excluding investments).   4. Health expenditure is for the insured population rather than resident population.

7.2.3 Total health expenditure as a share of GDP, 1995-2007

Selected OECD countries

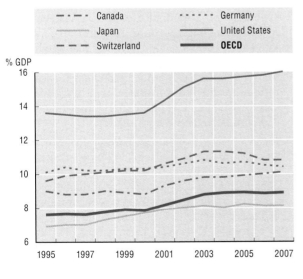

7.2.4 Total health expenditure per capita and GDP per capita, 2007

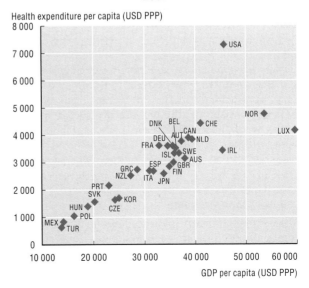

Source: OECD Health Data 2009.

StatLink ⬛⬛⬛ http://dx.doi.org/10.1787/720325225770

7.3. Health expenditure by function

The allocation of health spending across the different types of health services and medical goods is influenced by a range of factors, including the availability of resources such as hospital beds, physicians and access to new technology, the financial and institutional arrangements for health care delivery, as well as by national clinical guidelines and the disease burden within a country.

In 2007, curative and rehabilitative care provided in either an in-patient (including day care) or out-patient setting accounted for 60% of current health spending on average across OECD countries (Figure 7.3.1). The ratio of in-patient to out-patient spending depends on the institutional arrangements for health care provision. Austria and France, for example, report a relatively high proportion of expenditure for in-patient care (amounting to more than a third of total health spending) which is associated with a high level of hospital activity (see Indicator 4.4). Conversely, countries such as Portugal and Spain, with low levels of hospital activity, allocate less than a quarter of health care resources to in-patient care.

Large differences remain between countries in their expenditure on long-term care. Switzerland, Norway and Denmark, with established formal arrangements for elderly care, allocate up to a quarter of total health spending to long-term care. In Korea and Portugal, where care tends to be provided in more informal or family settings, the expenditure on long-term care occupies a much smaller share of total spending (OECD, 2005a).

The other major category of health expenditure is on medical goods, mostly accounted for by pharmaceuticals (see Indicator 7.4). Although over 20% on average, the share of health spending on medical goods can be as low as 11-13% in Luxembourg, Switzerland, Norway and Denmark, and as high as 36-38% in Hungary and the Slovak Republic.

Curative-rehabilitative care covers not only medical services requiring hospitalisation, but also those services provided either as day care, or as an out-patient in hospitals, the ambulatory sector, or in a patient's own home. Changes in medical practice, new technologies and more efficient allocation of resources can all affect the balance between different types of care delivery. Day (ambulatory) surgery is one area that has been expanding in many OECD countries in recent years.

The use of day surgery for procedures such as cataract removal (see Indicator 4.9) or hernia repairs may result in higher throughput and decreased unit costs. In many countries day care has accounted for an increasing share of the total spending on curative care in recent years (Figure 7.3.2). There are, however, wide variations in spending – partly reflecting data limitations – but also national policies and regulations. In France, spending on day care now accounts for around 11% of curative care spending. By contrast, Germany, where day surgery in public hospitals was prohibited until the late 1990s (Castoro et al., 2007), reported only 2% of curative care expenditure as services of day care.

Figure 7.3.3 shows the share of health expenditure allocated to public health and prevention activities. On average, OECD countries allocated 3% of their spending on health to a wide range of activities such as vaccination programmes and public health campaigns on alcohol abuse and smoking. The wide variation reflects to a great extent the national organisation of prevention campaigns. Where such initiatives are carried out at the primary care level, such as in Spain, the prevention function is not captured separately and may be included under the spending on curative care. Other countries adopting a more centralised approach to public health and prevention campaigns tend to be able to identify spending on such programmes.

Definition and deviations

The functional approach of the *System of Health Accounts* defines the boundaries of the health system. Total health expenditure consists of current health spending and investment. Current health expenditure comprises personal health care (curative care, rehabilitative care, long-term care, ancillary services and medical goods) and collective services (public health services and health administration). Curative, rehabilitative and long-term care can also be classified by mode of production (in-patient, day care, out-patient and home care.)

Factors limiting the comparability across countries include estimations of long-term care expenditure. Also, in some cases, expenditure in hospitals is used as a proxy for in-patient care services, although hospital expenditure may include spending on out-patient, ancillary, and in some cases drug dispensing services (Orosz and Morgan, 2004).

7.3.1 Current health expenditure by function of health care, 2007

Countries are ranked by in-patient curative care as a share of current expenditure on health

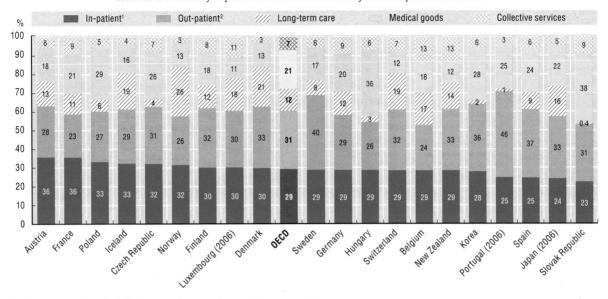

1. Refers to curative-rehabilitative care in in-patient and day-care settings.
2. Includes home-care and ancillary services

7.3.2 Day care as a share of total curative care expenditure, 2003 and 2007

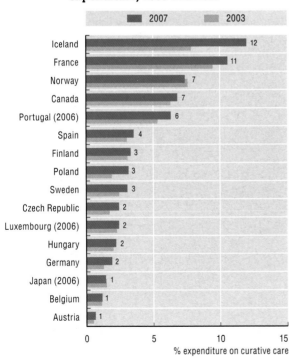

7.3.3 Expenditure on organised public health and prevention programmes, 2007

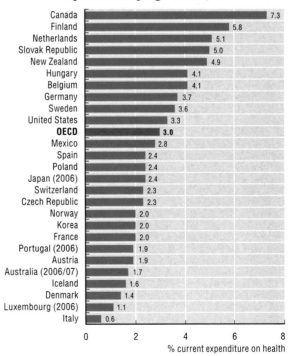

Source: OECD Health Data 2009.

StatLink http://dx.doi.org/10.1787/720355408522

Spending on pharmaceuticals accounts for a significant proportion of total health spending in OECD countries. Increased consumption of pharmaceuticals due to the diffusion of new drugs and the ageing of populations (see Indicator 4.10 "Pharmaceutical consumption") has been a major factor contributing to increased pharmaceutical expenditure and thus overall heath expenditure (OECD, 2008d). However, the relationship between pharmaceutical spending and total health spending is a complex one, in that increased expenditure on pharmaceuticals to tackle diseases may reduce the need for costly hospitalisation and intervention now or in the future.

The total pharmaceutical bill across OECD countries in 2007 is estimated to have reached more than USD 650 billion, accounting for around 15% of total health spending. Over the last ten years, average spending per capita on pharmaceuticals has risen by almost 50% in real terms. However, considerable variation in pharmaceutical spending can be observed, reflecting differences in volume, structure of consumption and pharmaceuticals pricing policies (Figure 7.4.1). In 2007, the United States spent the most per capita on pharmaceutical products, with spending of USD 878, compared with an OECD average of USD 461. The big pharmaceutical spenders after the United States were Canada and Greece. At the other end of the scale, Mexico spent just under USD PPP 200 per capita – less than a quarter of the US total. New Zealand and Poland also feature as one of the lowest per capita spenders at just over 50% of the OECD average. The low spending in New Zealand may be partly explained by a regulatory system that promotes the use of generics and the use of single supplier tenders to help reduce pharmaceutical prices (OECD, 2008d).

The public purse covers around 60% of pharmaceutical expenditure on average, much less than for physician and hospital services. This is due to higher co-payments for pharmaceuticals under public insurance schemes, or a lack of coverage for non-prescribed drugs and for prescribed drugs in some countries (see Table A.5 in Annex A for further information on basic primary health insurance coverage of selected health services and goods). The share of public expenditure for pharmaceutical drugs is the lowest in Mexico, at 21% in 2007, although it has increased over the past five years. In the United States and Canada, the public share is less than 40%, as private health insurance covers a large part of the bill. Public spending on prescription drugs in the United States increased in 2006, because of the introduction of the new Medicare drug programme for the elderly and the disabled. The public share of pharmaceutical spending increased from 24% in 2005 to 31% by 2007, but remains the second lowest share among OECD countries. At the other end of the scale, Greece, which has the highest private share of total health spending amongst the European countries, passes very little on in terms of user costs to the patient regarding pharmaceutical expenditure, with almost 80% funded out of public sources.

Pharmaceutical spending accounted for 1.5% of GDP on average across OECD countries, ranging from below 1% in countries such as Norway, Denmark and New Zealand, to more than 2% in Portugal, Greece, the Slovak Republic and Hungary (Figure 7.4.2).

Over the last ten years, the average growth in pharmaceutical spending has matched the growth in overall health spending, although different patterns emerge both between OECD countries and over time. Growth in pharmaceutical spending reached a peak in many countries between 1999 and 2001. Of the big pharmaceutical spenders, the United States and Canada have continued to see growth in pharmaceutical spending significantly above the average of OECD countries, although recent figures show lower growth rates (Figure 7.4.3). A number of countries have attempted to curb the relentless growth in pharmaceutical spending through such measures as the promotion of generic prescribing in the case of France (Fénina et al., 2008), or the introduction of cost sharing in the case of the Czech Republic (OECD, 2008a).

Definition and deviations

Pharmaceutical expenditure covers spending on prescription medicines and self-medication, often referred to as over-the-counter products, as well as other medical non-durable goods. It also includes pharmacists' remuneration when the latter is separate from the price of medicines. Pharmaceuticals consumed in hospitals are excluded. Final expenditure on pharmaceuticals includes wholesale and retail margins and value-added tax.

7.4.1 Expenditure on pharmaceuticals per capita, 2007

Public   Private

	USD PPP
United States	878
Canada	691
Greece	677
France	588
Belgium	566
Spain	562
Germany	542
Italy	518
Japan (2006)	506
Austria	500
Ireland	474
Portugal (2006)	468
OECD	**461**
Switzerland	454
Iceland	448
Sweden	446
Slovak Republic	435
Hungary	434
Australia (2006/07)	431
Netherlands	422
Korea	416
Finland	400
Norway	381
Czech Republic	349
Luxembourg[1]	338
Denmark	301
Poland	253
New Zealand	241
Mexico	198

1 000   800   600   400   200   0
USD PPP

1. Prescribed medicines only.

7.4.2 Expenditure on pharmaceuticals as share of GDP, 2007

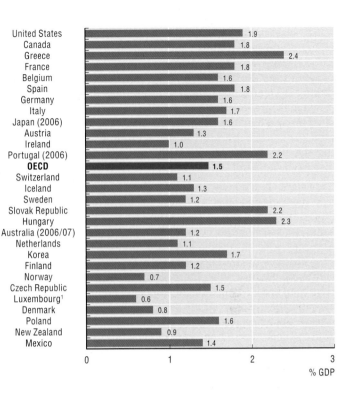

	% GDP
United States	1.9
Canada	1.8
Greece	2.4
France	1.8
Belgium	1.6
Spain	1.8
Germany	1.6
Italy	1.7
Japan (2006)	1.6
Austria	1.3
Ireland	1.0
Portugal (2006)	2.2
OECD	**1.5**
Switzerland	1.1
Iceland	1.3
Sweden	1.2
Slovak Republic	2.2
Hungary	2.3
Australia (2006/07)	1.2
Netherlands	1.1
Korea	1.7
Finland	1.2
Norway	0.7
Czech Republic	1.5
Luxembourg[1]	0.6
Denmark	0.8
Poland	1.6
New Zealand	0.9
Mexico	1.4

0   1   2   3
% GDP

7.4.3 Annual growth in pharmaceutical expenditure, 1997-2007

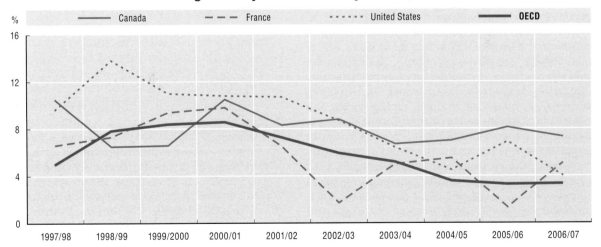

Canada —— France - - - United States ······· **OECD**

Source: OECD Health Data 2009.

StatLink ⚞ http://dx.doi.org/10.1787/720463218860

Attributing health care expenditure by disease and age is important for health policy makers in order to analyse resource allocations in the health care system. The information provided can play an important role in assessing the impact of ageing populations and changing disease patterns on spending. It can also provide input into the modelling of future health care expenditures (Heijink *et al.*, 2006). Furthermore, the linking of health expenditures by disease to appropriate measures of outputs (*e.g.* hospital discharges by disease) and outcomes (*e.g.* survival rates after heart attack or cancer) can provide useful input in monitoring the performance of health care systems at a disease-based level (AIHW, 2005).

Consistent "functionally defined" boundaries of health care spending and an accepted methodology for expenditure allocation are necessary for the production of comparative estimates of expenditure by disease. The data presented here come primarily from pilot studies in a number of OECD countries, supplemented by additional country data where similar methodologies have been used. There are significant data limitations in allocating health expenditure according to categories of disease, age and gender – especially in relation to household expenditure and out-patient categories. In order to maximize the comparability between countries, the figures provide a breakdown of hospital in-patient care – an area where administrative records are generally complete with the necessary diagnostic and patient information.

Figure 7.5.1 shows the distribution of hospital in-patient expenditure according to six main diagnostic categories. The countries show similar patterns, with circulatory diseases, cancers and mental and behavioural disorders accounting for close to 40% of total hospital in-patient expenditure. The differences between countries can be influenced by many factors, including demographic structure and disease patterns, as well as institutional arrangements and clinical guidelines for treating different diseases. Hungary allocates almost a quarter of hospital in-patient expenditure to the treatment of circulatory disease; this is not surprising since Hungary also reports the highest mortality rates among OECD countries due to ischaemic heart disease and stroke (see Indicator 1.4 "Mortality from heart disease and stroke"). Those countries allocating less to circulatory disease, such as Australia and France, also report lower mortality rates from such diseases.

The different cost patterns observed can be due to demographic factors. Figure 7.5.2 shows the relative allocation of hospital spending across three broad age groups. The share of hospital expenditure allocated to an age group is shown as a ratio to the size of that population. As expected, the population aged 65 and above consumes proportionally much more of hospital resources than those aged between 15-64. Australia and Korea allocate the greatest share of hospital expenditure to the elderly population. The organisation of care between different health care providers, particularly for the elderly population, is a significant factor in determining the level and share of hospital expenditure allocated between age groups. For example, the higher rates in Korea may be explained by the use of acute care beds for long-term care treatment (Hurst, 2007).

Figure 7.5.3 gives an indication of expenditure by hospital discharge for the two disease categories that consume the greatest share of hospital in-patient expenditure – circulatory disease and cancers. For circulatory disease, France, Germany and Sweden show the highest cost per discharge, while Sweden and Australia are highest for cancer treatment.

Definition and deviations

Expenditure by disease and age allocates current health expenditure by dimensions of patient characteristics. Guidelines currently being developed propose disease categories according to ICD-10 (with a mapping to ICD-9). Expenditures are also linked to one or more of the SHA dimensions of function (HC), provider (HP) and financing agent (HF). To ensure comparability between countries, a common methodology is proposed advocating primarily a top-down, main diagnostic allocation of expenditures.

The main comparability issues relate to the treatment of non-allocated and non-disease-specific expenditures. In the former case this is due to data limitations (often in out-patient and pharmaceutical expenditure) and in the latter case regarding some prevention and administration expenditure. For more meaningful comparisons a subset of expenditure can be used, such as in-patient care, where administrative records tend to be more complete.

7.5.1 Share of hospital in-patient spending by main diagnostic category, 2006

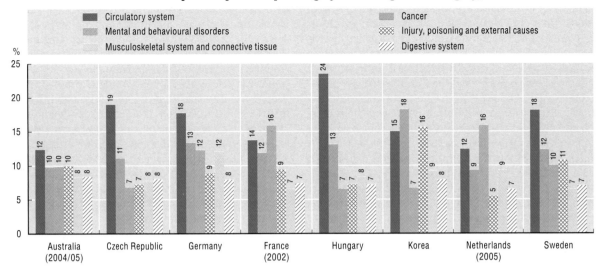

Note: Refers to share of total allocated expenditure. Czech Republic: Health Insurance Fund only. Germany: Total hospital expenditure. France: Curative care in hospitals. Hungary: Health Insurance and some local and central government expenditure. Netherlands: Curative care in general and specialty hospitals.

7.5.2 Relative hospital in-patient expenditure by age group

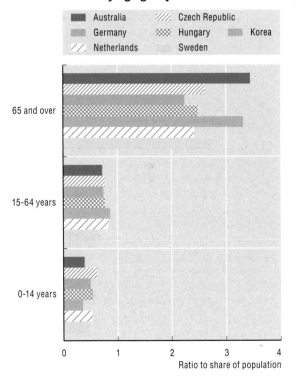

7.5.3 Expenditure per hospital discharge for two diagnostic categories

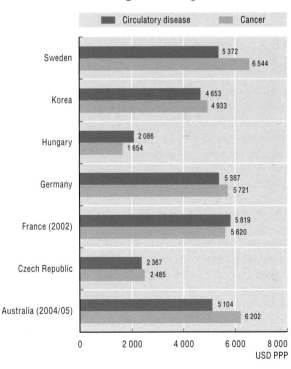

Source: Australia, Germany, Hungary, Korea and Sweden: OECD (2008), "Estimating Expenditure by Disease, Age and Gender under the System of Health Accounts (SHA) Framework"; Czech Republic: Unpublished data provided by Czech Statistical Office, May 2009; France: Fénina *et al.* (2006); Netherlands: Poos *et al.* (2008).

StatLink 🔢 http://dx.doi.org/10.1787/720474134843

7.6. Financing of health care

All OECD countries use a mix of public and private financing of health care, but to differing degrees. Public financing is confined to government revenues in countries where central and/or local governments are primarily responsible for financing health services directly (*e.g.* Spain and Norway). It comprises both general government revenues and social contributions in countries with social insurance based-funding (*e.g.* France and Germany). Private financing, on the other hand, covers households' out-of-pocket payments (either direct or as co-payments), third-party payment arrangements effected through various forms of private health insurance, health services such as occupational health care directly provided by employers, and other direct benefits provided by charities and the like.

Figure 7.6.1 shows the public share of health financing across OECD countries in 2007. The public sector is the main source of health financing in all OECD countries, apart from Mexico and the United States. On average, the public share of health spending was 73% in 2007, unchanged from 1990. In Luxembourg, the Czech Republic, the Nordic countries (except Finland), the United Kingdom, Japan, Ireland and New Zealand public financing accounted for more than 80% of all health expenditure. There has been a convergence of the public share of health spending among OECD countries over recent decades. Many of those countries with a relatively high public share in the early 1990s, such as Poland and Hungary, have decreased their share, while other countries which historically had a relatively low level (*e.g.* Portugal, Turkey) have increased their public share, reflecting health system reforms and the expansion of public coverage.

The fact that the health system is primarily public funded in most countries does not imply that the public sector plays the dominant role in every area of health care. Figure 7.6.2 shows the public share of financing separately for medical services and medical goods. The public sector plays a dominant role in paying for medical services in most countries (covering 78% on average), although a further sub-division of medical services shows an increasingly important role of private financing in the area of out-patient services (Orosz and Morgan, 2004), especially dental care, where around two-thirds of spending comes from private sources. In the financing of medical goods, private payments also play an important role, most clearly in Mexico, Canada, the United States and Poland.

The size and composition of private financing for all health services and goods differs considerably across countries. On average, more than two-thirds of private funding is accounted for by out-of-pocket payments (including any cost-sharing arrangements) (Colombo and Morgan, 2006). In some central and eastern European countries, the practice of unofficial supplementary payments means that the level of out-of-pocket spending is probably underestimated. Private health insurance is around 5-6% of total health expenditure on average across OECD countries (Figure 7.6.3). For some countries, it plays a significant financing role. It provides primary coverage for certain population groups in Germany, and for a large proportion of the non-elderly population in the United States, where private health insurance accounts for 35% of health expenditure. In France and Canada, private health insurance finances 13% of overall spending, but provides respectively complementary and supplementary coverage in a public system with universal reach (see Indicator 6.2).

In several countries, including the Netherlands and France, less than 2% of the total consumption of households was spent on out-of-pocket health services in 2007, while in Switzerland such spending represented more than 6% of total household consumption. In Korea and Mexico, it was 4-5% and the United States, with almost 3% of consumption being spent on out-of-pocket health services, was close to the OECD average.

Definition and deviations

There are three elements of health care financing: sources of funding (households, employers and the state), financing schemes (*e.g.* compulsory or voluntary insurance), and financing agents (organisations managing the financing schemes). Here "financing" is used in the sense of financing schemes as defined in the *System of Health Accounts*. Public financing includes general government revenues and social security funds. Private financing covers households' out-of-pocket payments, private health insurance and other private funds (NGOs and private corporations).

Out-of-pocket payments are expenditures borne directly by the patient. They include cost-sharing and, in certain countries, estimations of informal payments to health care providers.

7.6.1 Public share of total expenditure on health, 2007

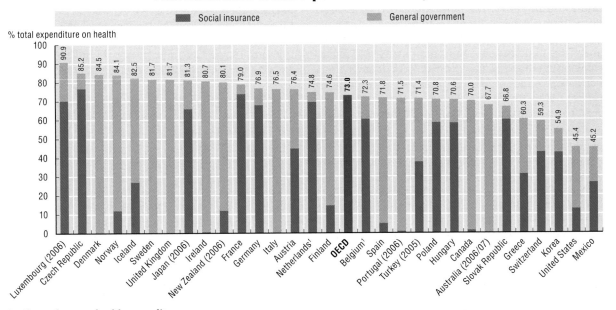

1. Share of current health expenditure.

7.6.2 Public share of expenditure on medical services and goods, 2007

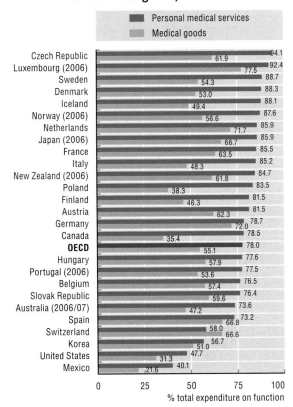

7.6.3 Out-of-pocket and private health insurance expenditure, 2007

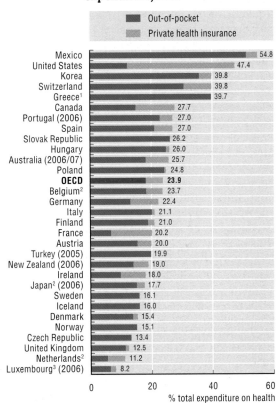

1. Total private expenditure. 2. Current expenditure. 3. Cost-sharing only.

Source: OECD Health Data 2009.

StatLink ⬛ᵢₛₘ http://dx.doi.org/10.1787/720482364801

International trade in health services and one of its main components, medical tourism, have been attracting increasing attention from health analysts, the medical profession, public health policy makers, and trade and tourism promotion agencies. Discussions on the opportunities and threats of such trade have been conducted with relatively little data to inform them.

The only reasonably comparable and widely reported measure of trade in health services is the balance of payments item "Health-related travel". This item is defined as "goods and services acquired by travellers going abroad travelling for medical reasons". This definition corresponds quite well to the notion of medical tourism. The concept has some limitations in that it does not include medical expenses of persons travelling for other reasons, and who happen to require medical services when abroad. Nor does it include health services provided cross-border such as medical laboratory services and telemedicine, or health services provided by medical personnel who go temporarily abroad. In the language of trade, exports of health-related travel from a reporting economy occur when domestic health service providers supply medical services to non-resident visitors travelling for medical reasons. Similarly, imports occur when residents of the reporting economy acquire medical services abroad from non-resident providers.

Data for around half of OECD countries shows that total reported exports and imports of health-related travel each amounted to about USD 5 billion in 2007. Due to definitional and measurement issues, this is a significant underestimate. Nevertheless, it is clear that, in comparison to the size of the health sector as a whole, medical tourism is marginal for most countries, but growing. In the case of Germany, reported health-related travel imports represent 0.5% of Germany's current health expenditure. However, from 2004 to 2007, they grew on average at 13% a year.

The United States is by far the largest exporter, reporting some USD 2.3 billion of exports in 2007 (Figure 7.7.1). The Czech Republic, Turkey, Belgium and Mexico all reported exports in excess of USD 300 million. Twenty-one OECD countries reported a total of USD 4.6 billion of health services imports, most in health-related travel in balance of payments sources and a few under the wider concept of imports of health care in the SHA data collection (Figure 7.7.2). Of these, Germany is by far the largest importer reporting some USD 1.5 billion of imports in 2007. The United States and Netherlands reported

imports of over USD 600 million, while Canada and Belgium reported imports above USD 300 million. The rate of growth of OECD imports of health-related travel was significantly higher than exports, suggesting the increasing importance of health services exported from non-OECD countries (Figures 7.7.3 and 7.7.4).

Despite increasing numbers of United States residents seeking treatment abroad, the United States remains a net exporter of medical services – with a USD 1.7 billion surplus in 2007. This export of health services includes visitors who suffer unexpected illness while in the United States (a wider definition than the one used in other countries), as well as international visitors, primarily from the Middle East, South America and Canada, coming with the express purpose of obtaining treatment. The motivations behind such inbound medical tourism can vary. For example, a number of medical institutions actively market their services to affluent consumers from emerging countries to come to the United States for specialised high quality care, or for services unavailable in their native countries. Some medical tourists may want to avoid extended waiting times within their home country. Other consumers may combine business or leisure travel with a specialised medical demand. Interestingly, the growth in exports slowed in 2007, due in part to the increased establishment of commercial hospitals abroad by US medical institutions (USITC, 2009).

Definition and deviations

According to the *Manual on Statistics of International Trade in Services*, "Health-related travel" is defined as "goods and services acquired by travellers going abroad for medical reasons". In the balance of payments, trade refers to goods and services transactions between residents and non-residents of an economy.

The *System of Health Accounts* includes imports within current health expenditure, defined as imports of medical goods and services for final consumption. Of these the purchase of medical services and goods, by resident patients while abroad, is currently the most important in value terms. This trade is not well reported by many of the countries reporting health accounts according to the SHA.

7.7.1 Exports of health-related travel, 2004 and 2007 (or nearest year)

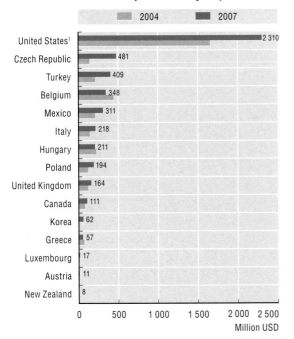

7.7.2 Imports of health-related travel, 2004 and 2007 (or nearest year)

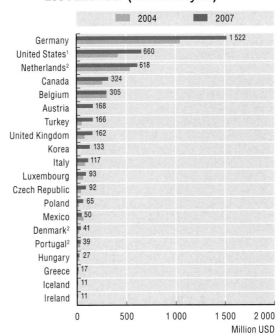

1. Expenditure by patients in foreign countries for treatment (BEA).   2. SHA concept of imports.

7.7.3 Annual average growth rate in health travel exports, 2004-07 (or nearest year)

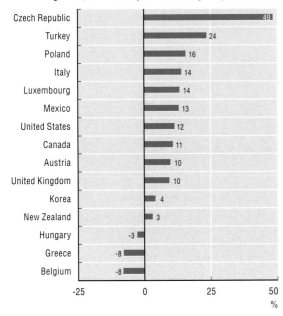

7.7.4 Annual average growth rate in health travel imports, 2004-07 (or nearest year)

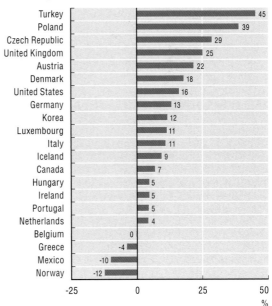

Note: Health-related travel exports occur when domestic providers supply medical services to non-residents travelling for medical reasons.

Source: OECD Statistics on International Trade in Services, IMF Balance of Payments Statistics, OECD System of Health Account.

StatLink ᥈᥈ᥔᥰ http://dx.doi.org/10.1787/720488885644

Bibliography

AAMC – Association of American Medical Colleges (2008), *The Complexities of Physician Supply and Demand: Projections through 2025*, Center for Workforce Studies, November.

Academy Health (2004), *Glossary of Terms Commonly Used in Health Care*, 2004 Edition, Washington DC.

ADA – American Diabetes Association (2008), "Economic Costs of Diabetes in the US in 2007", *Diabetes Care*, Vol. 31, No. 3, pp. 596-615.

AHRQ – Agency for Healthcare Research and Quality (2006), *Hospital and Ambulatory Surgery Care for Women's Cancers: HCUP Highlight*, No. 2, AHRQ, Rockville, MD.

AHRQ (2007a), *AHRQ Quality Indicators. Guide to Patient Safety Indicators. Version 3.1* (March 12, 2007), *www.qualityindicators.ahrq.gov/downloads/psi/psi_guide_v31.pdf*.

AHRQ (2007b), *Guide to Prevention Quality Indicators: Hospital Admissions for Ambulatory Care Sensitive Conditions*, AHRQ, Rockville, MD.

AHRQ (2008a), *2007 National Healthcare Disparities Report*, AHRQ, Rockville, MD.

AHRQ (2008b), *2007 National Healthcare Quality Report*, AHRQ, Rockville, MD.

AHRQ (2009), *Preventable Hospitalizations: Overview*, *www.ahrq.gov/data/hcup/factbk5/factbk5b.htm*.

AIHW – Australian Institute of Health and Welfare (2005), *Health System Expenditure on Disease and Injury in Australia 2000-01*, Second edition, AIHW, Canberra.

AIHW (2008a), *Breast Screen Australia Monitoring Report 2004-2005*, AIHW, Canberra.

AIHW (2008b), *Mental Health Services in Australia 2005-06*, AIHW, Canberra.

AIHW (2008c), *Rural, Regional and Remote Health: Indicators of Health System Performance*, AIHW, Canberra.

AIHW (2008d), *Diabetes: Australian Facts 2008*, AIHW, Canberra.

AIHW (2008e), *A Set of Performance Indicators across the Health and Aged Care System*, AIHW, Canberra.

Aiken, L. and R. Cheung (2008), "Nurse Workforce Challenges in the United States: Implications for Policy", *OECD Health Working Paper*, No. 35, OECD Publishing, Paris, October.

ALA – American Lung Association (2009), "Trends in Chronic Bronchitis and Emphysema: Morbidity and Mortality", *www.lungusa.org/site/c.dvLUK9O0E/b.252866/k.A435/COPD_Fact_Sheet.htm*, accessed on 20 August 2009.

Allin, S. (2006), "Equity in the Use of Health Services in Canada and its Provinces", LSE Health Working Paper, No. 3/2006, London School of Economics and Political Science, London.

Anderson G.F. and B.K. Frogner (2008), "Health Spending in OECD Countries: Obtaining Value per Dollar", *Health Affairs*, Vol. 27, No. 6, pp. 1718-1726.

Antonazzo, E. et al. (2003), "The Labour Market for Nursing: A Review of the Labour Supply Literature", *Health Economics*, Vol. 12, pp. 465-478.

Arah, O. et al. (2006), "A Conceptual Framework for the OECD Health Care Quality Indicators Project", *International Journal for Quality in Health Care*, Vol. 18, Supplement 1, pp. 5-13.

Baker, L., S.W. Atlas and C.C. Afendulis (2008), "Expanded Use of Imaging Technology and the Challenge of Measuring Value", *Health Affairs*, Vol. 27, No. 6, pp. 1467-1478.

Banthin, J.S., P. Cunningham and D.M. Bernard (2008), "Financial Burden of Health Care, 2001-2004", *Health Affairs*, Vol. 27, pp. 188-195.

Beck, L.F., A.M. Dellinger and M.E. O'Neil (2007), "Motor Vehicle Crash Injury Rates by Mode of Travel, United States: Using Exposure-based Methods to Quantify Differences", *American Journal of Epidemiology*, Vol. 166, pp. 212-218.

Belizán, J.M. *et al.* (1999), "Rates and Implications of Caesarean Sections in Latin America: Ecological Analysis", *BMJ*, Vol. 319, pp. 1397-1400.

Bellanger, M. and Z. Or (2008), "What Can We Learn From a Cross-Country Comparison of the Costs of Child Delivery?", *Health Economics*, Vol. 17, pp. S47-S57.

Bennett, J. (2003), "Investment in Population Health in Five OECD Countries", OECD Health Working Paper, No. 2, OECD Publishing, Paris.

Bewley, S. and J. Cockburn (2002), "The Unethics of 'Request' Caesarean Section", *BJOG: An International Journal of Obstetrics and Gynaecology*, Vol. 109, pp. 593-596.

Blendon, R. *et al.* (2002), "Inequalities in Health Care: A Five-Country Survey", *Health Affairs*, Vol. 21, pp. 182-191.

BOLD Collaborative Research Group (2007), "International Variation in the Prevalence of COPD (The BOLD Study): A Population-Based Prevalence Study", *The Lancet*, Vol. 370, pp. 741-750.

Bourgueil, Y., A. Marek and J. Mousquès (2006), "Vers une coopération entre médecins et infirmières – l'apport d'expériences européennes et canadiennes", DREES, Série études, No. 57, March.

Brandt, N. (2008), "Moving Towards More Sustainable Healthcare Financing in Germany", OECD Economics Department Working Paper, No. 612, OECD Publishing, Paris.

Brown, M.L. *et al.* (2002), "Estimating Health Care Costs Related to Cancer Treatment from SEER-Medicare Data", *Medical Care*, Vol. 40, No. 8, pp. IV-104-117.

Burns, A., D. van der Mensbrugghe and H. Timmer (2008), *Evaluating the Economic Consequences of Avian Influenza*, World Bank, Washington.

Busse, R. and A. Riesberg (2004), *Health Care Systems in Transition: Germany*, WHO Regional Office for Europe on behalf of the European Observatory on Health Systems and Policies, Copenhagen.

Cartera, K.N. *et al.* (2007), "Improved Survival after Stroke: Is Admission to Hospital the Major Explanation? Trend Analyses of the Auckland Regional Community Stroke Studies", *Cerebrovascular Diseases*, Vol. 23, pp. 162-168.

Cash, R. and P. Ulmann (2008), "Projet OCDE sur la migration des professionnels de santé : Le cas de la France" (OECD project on the migration of health professionals: The case of France), OECD Health Working Paper, No. 36, OECD Publishing, Paris, October.

Castoro, C. *et al.* (2007), *Policy Brief-Day Surgery: Making it Happen*, World Health Organisation on Behalf of the European Observatory on Health Systems and Policies, Copenhagen.

CCCG – Colorectal Cancer Collaborative Group (2000), "Palliative Chemotherapy for Advanced Colorectal Cancer: Systematic Review and Meta-analysis", *British Medical Journal*, Vol. 321, pp. 531-535.

CDC – Centers for Disease Control and Prevention (2008), *Factsheet: HIV/AIDS in the United States*, US National Center for Health Statistics.

CDC (2009a), "Births: Preliminary Data for 2007", *National Vital Statistics Reports*, Vol. 57, No. 11, US National Center for Health Statistics.

CDC (2009b), "Key Facts About Seasonal Influenza (Flu)", *www.cdc.gov/flu/keyfacts.htm*, accessed on 20 August 2009.

Ceia, F. *et al.* (2002), "Prevalence of Chronic Heart Failure in South-Western Europe: The EPICA study", *European Journal of Heart Failure*, Vol. 4, pp. 531-539.

Chaloff, J. (2008), "Mismatches in the Formal Sector, Expansion of the Informal Sector: Immigration of Health Professionals to Italy", OECD Health Working Paper, No. 34, OECD Publishing, Paris.

Chiha, Y.A. and C.R. Link (2003), "The Shortage of Registered Nurses and Some New Estimates of the Effects of Wages on Registered Nurses Labour Supply: A Look at the Past and a Preview of the 21st Century", *Health Policy*, Vol. 64, pp. 349-375.

CIBIS-II Investigators and Committees (1999), "The Cardiac Insufficiency Bisoprolol Study II (CIBIS-II): A Randomised Trial", *The Lancet*, Vol. 353, pp. 9-13.

CIHI – Canadian Institute for Health Information (2005), *Geographic Distribution of Physicians in Canada: Beyond How Many and Where*, CIHI, Ottawa.

CIHI (2007), "Trends in Acute Inpatient Hospitalisations and Day Surgery Visits in Canada, 1995-1996 to 2005-2006", *Analysis in Brief*, CIHI, Ottawa.

CIHI (2008a), *Medical Imaging in Canada, 2007*, CIHI, Ottawa.

CIHI (2008b), *Workforce Trends of Pharmacists for Selected Provinces and Territories in Canada, 2007*, CIHI, Ottawa.

CIHI (2009), *Health Indicators 2009*, CIHI, Ottawa.

Cleland, J.G. *et al.* (2003), "The EuroHeart Failure Survey Programme: A Survey on the Quality of Care among Patients with Heart Failure in Europe. Part 1: Patient Characteristics and Diagnosis", *European Heart Journal*, Vol. 24, No. 5, pp. 442-463.

Cole, T.J. *et al.* (2000), "Establishing a Standard Definition for Child Overweight and Obesity Worldwide: International Survey", *British Medical Journal*, Vol. 320, pp. 1-6.

Coleman, M.P. *et al.* (2008), "Cancer Survival in Five Continents: A Worldwide Population-Based Study (CONCORD)", *Lancet Oncol*, Vol. 9, pp. 730-756.

Colombo, F. and D. Morgan (2006), "Evolution of Health Expenditure in OECD Countries", *Revue française des affaires sociales*, April-September.

Commonwealth Fund (2008), *National Scorecard on US Health System Performance, 2008*, Chartpack, Commonwealth Fund, New York.

Council of the European Union (2009), *Council Recommendation on Patient Safety, Including the Prevention and Control of Healthcare Associated Infections*, No. 10120/09, Brussels, June.

Couture, M.C. *et al.* (2008), "Inequalities in Breast and Cervical Cancer Screening among Urban Mexican Women", *Preventive Medicine*, Vol. 47, pp. 471-476.

Currie, C. *et al.* (eds.) (2000), *Health and Health Behaviour among Young People (1997/98)*, WHO Regional Office for Europe, Copenhagen.

Currie, C. *et al.* (eds.) (2004), *Young People's Health in Context: International Report from the HBSC 2001/2002 Survey*, WHO Regional Office for Europe, Copenhagen.

Currie, C. *et al.* (eds.) (2008), *Inequalities in Young People's Health: Health Behaviour in School-aged Children (HBSC) International Report from the 2005/2006 Survey*, WHO Regional Office for Europe, Copenhagen.

Cutler, D. and E.L. Glaeser (2006), "Why do Europeans Smoke More Than Americans?", Working Paper, No. 12124, National Bureau of Economic Research, Cambridge, MA.

Dartmouth Atlas of Health Care (2005), "Studies of Surgical Variation, Cardiac Surgery Report", *www.dartmouthatlas.org/index.shtm*.

Davies, M. *et al.* (2001), "Prevalence of Left-Ventricular Systolic Dysfunction and Heart Failure in the Echocardiographic Heart of England Screening Study: A Population-Based Study", *The Lancet*, Vol. 358, pp. 439-444.

Davis, K. *et al.* (2007), "Mirror, Mirror on the Wall: An International Update on the Comparative Performance of American Health Care", Commonwealth Fund, New York.

De Graeve, D. and T. Van Ourti (2003), "The Distributional Impact of Health Financing in Europe: A Review", *The World Economy*, Vol. 26, pp. 459-1479.

de Looper, M. and G. Lafortune (2009), "Measuring Disparities in Health Status and in Access and Use of Health Care in OECD Countries", OECD Health Working Paper, No. 43, OECD Publishing, Paris, March.

Declercq, E., F. Menacker and M. Macdorman (2005), "Rise in 'No Indicated Risk' Primary Caesareans in the United States, 1991-2001: Cross Sectional Analysis", *British Medical Journal*, Vol. 330, pp. 71-72.

Department of Health and Children (2001), "National Health Strategy: Quality and Fairness – A Health System for You", Stationery Office, Dublin.

Di Mario, S. *et al.* (2005), *What is the Effectiveness of Antenatal Care? (Supplement)*, WHO Regional Office for Europe (Health Evidence Network Report), Copenhagen.

Diabetes Control and Complications Trial Research Group (1996), "Lifetime Benefits and Costs of Intensive Therapy as Practiced in the Diabetes Control and Complications Trial", *Journal of the American Medical Association*, Vol. 276, pp. 725-734.

DREES – Direction de la recherche, des études, de l'évaluation et des statistiques (2007), "Les chirurgiens-dentistes en France", *Études et résultats*, No. 594, Paris, September.

DREES (2008), "Les médecins – Estimations au 1er janvier 2008", Document de travail, No. 127, Paris.

DREES (2009), "La démographie médicale à l'horizon 2030 : de nouvelles projections nationales et régionales", *Études et résultats*, No. 679, February.

Drösler, S.E. (2008), "Facilitating Cross-National Comparisons of Indicators for Patient Safety at the Health-System Level in the OECD Countries", OECD Health Technical Paper, No. 19, OECD Publishing, Paris.

Drösler, S.E. *et al.* (2009a), "Application of Patient Safety Indicators Internationally: A Pilot Study among Seven Countries", *International Journal of Quality in Health Care*, Vol. 21, pp. 272-278.

Drösler, S.E. *et al.* (2009b), "Health Care Quality Indicators Project, Patient Safety Indicators Report 2009", OECD Health Working Paper, forthcoming, OECD Publishing, Paris.

Dumont, J.C., P. Zurn, J. Church and C. Le Thi (2008), "International Mobility of Health Professionals and Health Workforce Management in Canada: Myths and Realities", OECD Health Working Paper, No. 40, OECD Publishing, Paris.

Eagle, K.A. *et al.* (2005), "Guideline-Based Standardized Care is Associated with Substantially Lower Mortality in Medicare Patients with Acute Myocardial Infarction: The American College of Cardiology's Guidelines Applied in Practice (GAP)", *J Am Coll Cardiol*, Vol. 46, pp. 1242-1248.

Ebihara, S. (2007), "More Doctors Needed Before Boosting Clinical Research in Japan", *The Lancet*, Vol. 369, No. 9579, p. 2076.

ECDC (European Centre for Disease Prevention and Control) and WHO Regional Office for Europe (2008), *HIV/AIDS Surveillance in Europe 2007*, ECDC, Stockholm.

Eder, W., M. Ege and E. von Mutius (2006), "The Asthma Epidemic", *NEJM*, Vol. 355, No. 21, pp. 2226-2235.

ETSC – European Transport Safety Council (2003), *Transport Safety Performance in the EU: A Statistical Overview*, ETSC, Brussels.

Eurobarometer (2006), "Mental Well-being, Special Eurobarometer 248/Wave 64.4", May.

EUROCARE Working Group (2007), "Trends in Cervical Cancer Survival in Europe, 1983-1994: A Population-Based Study", *Gynecologic Oncology*, Vol. 105, No. 3, pp. 609-619.

European Commission (2006), *European Guidelines for Quality Assurance in Breast Cancer Screening and Diagnosis*, 4th edition, Luxembourg.

European Commission (2008a), *Hospital Data Project Phase 2*, Final Report, Luxembourg, November.

European Commission (2008b), *Major and Chronic Diseases-Report 2007*, EC Directorate-General for Health and Consumers, Luxembourg.

European Commission (2008c), *European Guidelines for Quality Assurance in Cervical Cancer Screening*, 2nd edition, Luxembourg.

European Union (2003), "Council Recommendation of 2 December 2003 on cancer screening (2003/879/EC)", *Official Journal of the European Union*, L327, Vol. 46, 16 December 2003, pp. 34-38.

Euro-Peristat (2008), *European Perinatal Health Report, 2008*, Luxembourg.

Faivre-Finn, C. *et al.* (2002), "Colon Cancer in France: Evidence for Improvement in Management and Survival", *Gut*, Vol. 51, No. 1, pp. 60-64.

Fedorowicz, Z., D. Lawrence and P. Gutierrez (2004), "Day Care *versus* In-patient Surgery for Age-related Cataract", *Cochrane Database of Systematic Reviews*, Vol. 25, No. CD004242.

Fénina, A. *et al.* (2006), "Les dépenses de prévention et les dépenses de soins par pathologie en France", *Questions d'économie de la santé*, No. 111, July.

Fénina, A, Y. Geffroy and M. Duée (2008), "Comptes nationaux de la santé, 2007", Document de travail, Série statistiques, No. 126, Direction de la recherche, des études, de l'évaluation et des statistiques (DREES), Paris, September.

Feuer, E.J. *et al.* (2003), "The Lifetime Risk of Developing Breast Cancer", *www.srab.cancer.gov/devcan/report1.pdf*.

FHF – Fédération hospitalière de France (2008), *Étude sur les césariennes*, FHF, Paris.

Foresight (2007), "Tackling Obesities: Future Choices", Government Office for Science, *www.foresight.gov.uk/Obesity/17.pdf*.

Fox, K.A.A. *et al.* (2007), "Declines in Rates of Death and Heart Failure in Acute Coronary Syndromes, 1999-2006", *JAMA*, Vol. 297, No. 17, pp. 1892-1900.

Fujisawa, R. and G. Lafortune (2008), "The Remuneration of General Practitioners and Specialists in 14 OECD Countries: What are the Factors Explaining Variations Across Countries", OECD Health Working Paper, No. 41, OECD Publishing, December.

Gakidou, E., S. Nordhagen and Z. Obermeyer (2008), "Coverage of Cervical Cancer Screening in 57 Countries: Low Average Levels and Large Inequalities", PLoS Medicine, Vol. 5, No. 6, pp. 0863-0868.

Garcia Armesto, S., M.L. Gil Lapetra, L. Wei, E. Kelley et al. (2007), "Health Care Quality Indicators Project 2006 Data Collection Update Report", OECD Health Working Paper, No. 29, OECD Publishing, Paris.

Garcia Armesto, S., H. Medeiros and L. Wei (2008), "Information Availability for Measuring and Comparing Quality of Mental Health Care across OECD Countries", OECD Health Technical Paper, No. 20, OECD Publishing, Paris.

Gatta, G., M.B. Lasota, A. Verdecchia and the EUROCARE Working Group (1998), "Survival of European Women with Gynaecological Tumours, during the Period 1978-1989", European Journal of Cancer, Vol. 34, No. 14, pp. 2218-2225.

Gatta, G. et al. (2000), "Toward a Comparison of Survival in American and European Cancer Patients", Cancer, Vol. 89, No. 4, pp. 893-900.

Gil, M., J. Marrugat and J. Sala (1999), "Relationship of Therapeutic Improvements and 28-day Case Fatality in Patients Hospitalized with Acute Myocardial Infarction between 1978 and 1993 in the REGICOR Study, Gerona, Spain", Circulation, Vol. 99, pp. 1767-1773.

Goldberg, R.J., J. Yaerzebski and D. Lessard (1999), "A Two-decades (1975 to 1995) Long Experience in the Incidence, In-hospital and Long-term Case-fatality Rates of Acute Myocardial Infarction: A Community-wide Perspective", Journal of the American College of Cardiology, Vol. 33, pp. 1533-1539.

Govindarajan, A. et al. (2006), "Population-based Assessment of the Surgical Management of Locally Advanced Colorectal Cancer", Journal of the National Cancer Institute, Vol. 98, pp. 1474-1481.

Greenfield, S., A. Nicolucci and S. Mattke (2004), "Selecting Indicators for the Quality of Diabetes Care at the Health Systems Level in OERCD Countries", OECD Health Technical Paper, No. 15, OECD Publishing, Paris.

Hacke, W. et al. (1995), "Intravenous Thrombolysis with Recombinant Tissue Plasminogen Activator for Acute Hemispheric Stroke. The European Co-operative Acute Stroke Study (ECASS)", Journal of the American Medical Association, Vol. 274, No. 13, pp. 1017-1025.

Haffner, S.M. (2000), "Coronary Heart Disease in Patients with Diabetes", New England Journal of Medicine, Vol. 342, pp. 1040-1042.

Hajjar, I., J.M. Kotchen and T.A. Kotchen (2006), "Hypertension: Trends in Prevalence, Incidence, and Control", Annual Review of Public Health, Vol. 27, pp. 465-490.

Hallal, P.C. et al. (2006), "Adolescent Physical Activity and Health: A Systematic Review", Sports Medicine, Vol. 36, No. 12, pp. 1019-1030.

Harper, D.M. et al. (2006), "Sustained Efficacy up to 4-5 Years of a Bivalent L1 Virus-like Particle Vaccine against Human Papillomavirus Types 16 and 18: Follow-up from Randomised Control Trial", The Lancet, Vol. 367, pp. 1247-1255.

Hasselhorn, H.M., B.H. Muller and G.P. Tackenber (2005), NEXT Scientific Report, University of Wuppertal, Wuppertal.

Hawton, K. and K. van Heeringen (2009), "Suicide", The Lancet, Vol. 373, pp. 1373-1381.

Heijink, R., M.A. Koopmanschap and J.J. Polder (2006), International Comparison of Cost of Illness, RIVM, Bilthoven.

Hermann, R., S. Mattke et al. (2004), "Selecting Indicators for the Quality of Mental Health Care at the Health Systems Level in OECD Countries", OECD Health Technical Paper, No. 17, OECD Publishing, Paris.

HHS – Health and Human Services (2004), The Health Consequences of Smoking: A Report of the Surgeon General, DHHS, Washington DC.

HHS Office of Health Reform (2009), "Health Disparities: A Case for Closing the Gap", US Department of Health and Human Services, www.healthreform.gov.

Hisashige, A. (1992), "The Introduction and Evaluation of MRI in Japan", International Society for Technology Assessment in Health Care, Vol. 3, No. 126.

Hockley, T. and M. Gemmill (2007), *European Cholesterol Guidelines Report*, Policy Analysis Centre, London School of Economics, London.

Hoffman, C., D. Rowland and E.C. Hamel (2005), *Medical Debt and Access to Health Care*, Kaiser Commission on Medicaid and the Uninsured, Washington, September.

HRSA – Health Resources and Services Administration (2004), *What is behind HRSA's Projected Supply, Demand and Shortage of Registered Nurses?*, HRSA, Rockville, MD.

Huang, C.M. (2008), "Human Papillomavirus and Vaccination", *Mayo Clinic Proceedings*, Vol. 83, No. 6, pp. 701-707.

Huber, M., A. Stanicole, J. Bremner and K. Wahlbeck (2008), *Quality in and Equality of Access to Healthcare Services*, European Commission Directorate-General for Employment, Social Affairs and Equal Opportunities, Luxembourg.

Hurst, J. (2007), "Towards a Sustainable Health and Long-term Care Policy", *Facing the Future: Korea's Family, Pension and Health Policy Challenges*, OECD Publishing, Paris.

IARC – International Agency for Research on Cancer (2004), "GLOBOCAN 2002: Cancer Incidence, Mortality and Prevalence Worldwide", *IARC CancerBase*, No. 5, Version 2.0, IARC Press, Lyon.

IARC (2008), *World Cancer Report 2008*, IARC Press, Lyon.

IDF – International Diabetes Federation (2006), *Diabetes Atlas*, 3rd edition, IDF, Brussels.

IDF (2009), *Diabetes Atlas*, 4th edition, IDF, Brussels.

IHE – Institute of Health Economics (2008), *Determinants and Prevention of Low Birth Weight: A Synopsis of the Evidence*, IHE, Alberta, Canada.

IMA-AIM – Intermutualistisch Agentschap (2009), "Programma Borstkankerscreening, Vergelijking van de Eerste Drie Rondes, 2001-2002, 2003-2004 en 2005-2006", Brussels.

Institute of Alcohol Studies (2007), "Binge Drinking-Nature, Prevalence and Causes", *IAS Fact Sheet*, *www.ias.org.uk/resources/factsheets/binge_drinking.pdf*.

Institute of Cancer Research (2009), "Prostate Cancer", *Fact Sheet, www.icr.ac.uk/everyman/about/prostate.html*.

Jadwiga, A. Wedzicha and T.A.R. Seemungal (2007), "COPD Exacerbations: Defining their Cause and Prevention", *The Lancet*, Vol. 370, pp. 786-796.

Japanese Nursing Association (2009), *Nursing Statistics, www.nurse.or.jp/jna/english/statistics/index.html*.

Japanese Pharmaceutical Association (2008), *Annual Report of JPA 2008-2009*, JPA, Tokyo.

Jha, P. *et al.* (2006), "Social Inequalities in Male Mortality, and in Male Mortality from Smoking: Indirect Estimation from National Death Rates in England and Wales, Poland, and North America", *The Lancet*, Vol. 368, No. 9533, pp. 367-370.

Johanson, R. (2002), "Has the Medicalisation of Childbirth Gone Too Far?", *British Medical Journal*, Vol. 324, No. 7342, pp. 892-895.

Joumard, I., C. Andre, C. Nicq and O. Chatal (2008), "Health Status Determinants: Lifestyle, Environment, Health Care Resources and Efficiency", *Economics Department Working Paper*, No. 627, OECD Publishing, Paris.

Kaikkonen, R. (2007), *TEROKA-Project for Reducing Socioeconomic Health Inequalities in Finland*, Ministry of Social Affairs and Health, *www.teroka.fi*.

Kearney, P. *et al.* (2005), "Global Burden of Hypertension: Analysis of Worldwide Data", *The Lancet*, Vol. 365, No. 9455, pp. 217-223.

Keech, M., A.J. Scott and P.J. Ryan (1998), "The Impact of Influenza and Influenza-like Illness on Productivity and Healthcare Resource Utilization in a Working Population", *Occupational Medicine*, Vol. 49, pp. 85-90.

Kelley, E. and J. Hurst (2006), "Health Care Quality Indicators Project Conceptual Framework", *OECD Health Working Paper*, No. 23, OECD Publishing, Paris.

Khush, K.K., E. Rapaport and D. Waters (2005), "The History of the Coronary Care Unit", *Canadian Journal of Cardiology*, Vol. 21, pp. 1041-1045.

Kiely, J., K. Brett, S. Yu and D. Rowley (1995), "Low Birth Weight and Intrauterine Growth Retardation", in L. Wilcox and J. Marks (eds.), *From Data to Action: CDC's Public Health Surveillance for Women, Infants, and Children*, Center for Disease Control and Preventions, Atlanta, pp. 185-202.

King, H., R.E. Aubert and W.H. Herman (1998), "Global Burden of Diabetes, 1995-2025: Prevalence, Numerical Estimates, and Projections", *Diabetes Care*, Vol. 21, No. 9, pp. 1414-1431.

Komajda, M. *et al.* (2003), "The EuroHeart Failure Survey Programme: A Survey on the Quality of Care among Patients with Heart Failure in Europe. Part 2: Treatment", *European Heart Journal*, Vol. 24, No. 5, pp. 464-474.

Kovess-Masfety, V. *et al.* (2007), "Differences in Lifetime Use of Services for Mental Health Problems in Six European Countries", *Psychiatric Services*, Vol. 58, No. 2, pp. 213-220.

Kunze, U. *et al.* (2007), "Influenza Vaccination in Austria, 1982-2003", *Wien Med Wochenschr*, Vol. 157, No. 5-6, pp. 98-101.

Kwon, J.-K., H. Chun and S. Cho (2009), "A Closer Look at the Increase in Suicide Rates in South Korea from 1986-2005", *BMC Public Health*, Vol. 9, No. 72.

Lafortune, G., G. Balestat *et al.* (2007), "Trends in Severe Disability among Elderly People: Assessing the Evidence in 12 OECD Countries and Future Implications", OECD Health Working Paper, No. 26, OECD Publishing, Paris.

Lagrew, D.C. and J.A. Adashek (1998), "Lowering the Cesarean Section Rate in a Private Hospital: Comparison of Individual Physicians' Rates, Risk Factors and Outcomes", *Am J Obstet Gynecol*, Vol. 178, pp. 1207-1214.

Lambie, L., S. Mattke *et al.* (2004), "Selecting Indicators for the Quality of Cardiac Care at the Health Systems Level in OECD Countries", OECD Health Technical Paper, No. 14, OECD Publishing, Paris.

Laws, P.J. and L. Hilder (2008), *Australia's Mothers and Babies 2006*, AIHW National Perinatal Statistics Unit, Sydney.

Lee, W.C., Y.E. Chavez *et al.* (2004), "Economic Burden of Heart Failure: A Summary of Recent Literature", *Heart and Lung*, Vol. 33, No. 6, pp. 362-371.

Lien, L. (2002), "Are Readmission Rates Influenced by How Psychiatric Services are Organized?", *Nordic Journal of Psychiatry*, Vol. 56, pp. 23-28.

Lu, J.R. *et al.* (2007), "Horizontal Equity in Health Care Utilization Evidence from Three High-income Asian Economies", *Social Science and Medicine*, Vol. 64, pp. 199-212.

Mackenbach, J.P. *et al.* (2008), "Socioeconomic Inequalities in Health in 22 European Countries", *New England Journal of Medicine*, Vol. 358, pp. 2468-2481.

Mackie, C.O. *et al.* (2009), "Hepatitis B Immunisation Strategies: Timing is Everything", *CMAJ*, Vol. 18, No. 2, pp. 196-202.

Marshall, M. *et al.* (2004), "Selecting Indicators for the Quality of Health Promotion, Prevention and Primary Care at the Health Systems Level in OECD Countries", OECD Health Technical Paper, No. 16, OECD Publishing, Paris.

Masoli, M., D. Fabian, S. Holt and R. Beasley (2004), *Global Burden of Asthma*, Global Initiative for Asthma.

Mathers, C. *et al.* (2005), "Counting the Dead and What They Died From: An Assessment of the Global Status of Cause of Death Data", *Bulletin of the World Health Organisation*, Vol. 83, No. 3, pp. 171-177, March.

Mattke, S., E. Kelley, P. Scherer, J. Hurst, M.-L. Gil Lapetra *et al.* (2006), "Health Care Quality Indicators Project Initial Indicators Report", OECD Health Working Paper, No. 22, OECD Publishing, Paris.

Mauri, D., N.P. Polyzos *et al.* (2008), "Multiple-Treatments Meta-Analysis of Chemotherapy and Targeted Therapies in Advanced Breast Cancer", *Journal of the National Cancer Institute*, Vol. 100, No. 24, pp. 1745-1747.

McGlynn, E.A. *et al.* (2003), "The Quality of Health Care Delivered to Adults in the United States", *New England Journal of Medicine*, Vol. 348, No. 26, pp. 2635-2645.

Melander, A. *et al.* (2006), "Utilisation of Antihyperglycaemic Drugs in Ten European Countries: Different Developments and Different Levels", *Diabetologia*, Vol. 49, pp. 2024-2029.

Miilunpalo, S. *et al.* (1997), "Self-rated Health Status as a Health Measure: The Predictive Value of Self-reported Health Status on the Use of Physician Services and on Mortality in the Working-age Population", *Journal of Clinical Epidemiology*, Vol. 50, pp. 90-93.

Miller, A. (2006), "The Impact of Midwifery-Promoting Public Policies on Medical Interventions and Health Outcomes", *Advances in Economic Analysis and Policy*, Vol. 6, No. 1, pp. 1-34.

Ministry of Health (2007), *Health Targets: Moving towards Healthier Futures 2007/2008*, Ministry of Health, Wellington.

Minkoff, H. and F.A. Chervenak (2003), "Elective Primary Cesarean Section", *New England Journal of Medicine*, Vol. 348, pp. 946-950.

Moïse, P. (2003), "The Heart of the Health Care System: Summary of the Ischaemic Heart Disease Part of the OECD Ageing-related Diseases Study", *A Disease-based Comparison of Health Systems: What is Best and at What Cost?*, OECD Publishing, Paris.

Moïse, P. et al. (2003), "OECD Study of Cross-national Differences in the Treatment, Costs and Outcomes for Ischaemic Heart Disease", OECD Health Working Paper, No. 3, OECD Publishing, Paris.

Moon, L. et al. (2003), "Stroke Care in OECD Countries: A Comparison of Treatment, Costs and Outcomes in 17 OECD Countries", OECD Health Working Paper, No. 5, OECD Publishing, Paris.

Moorman, J.E. et al. (2007), "National Surveillance for Asthma – United States, 1980-2004", *MMWR Surveill Summ*, Vol. 56, No. 8, pp. 1-54.

Mori, E. et al. (1992), "Intravenous Recombinant Tissue Plasminogen Activator in Acute Carotid Artery Territory Stroke", *Neurology*, Vol. 42, No. 5, pp. 976-982.

National Board of Health and Welfare (2008), *Quality and Efficiency in Swedish Health Care – Regional Comparisons 2008*, Stockholm.

National Heart Foundation of Australia and the Cardiac Society of Australia and New-Zealand (2005), "Position Statement on Lipid Management-2005".

NCHS – National Centre for Health Statistics (2007), *Health, United States, 2007*, NCHS, Hyattsville, MD.

NCHS (2009), *Health, United States, 2008*, NCHS, Hyattsville, MD.

NHSBSP – National Health Service Breast Screening Programme (2008), *NHS Breast Screening Programme, Annual Review 2008*, London.

Nicholson, K.G., R. Snacken and A.M. Palache (1995), "Influenza Immunization Policies in Europe and the United States", *Vaccine*, Vol. 13, No. 4, pp. 365-369.

NINDS – National Institute of Neurological Disorders and Stroke (1995), "Tissue Plasminogen Activator for Acute Ischemic Stroke", *New England Journal of Medicine*, Vol. 333, No. 24, pp. 1581-1587.

NOMESCO (2004), "Equal Access to Care", *Health Statistics in the Nordic Countries 2002*, NOMESCO, Copenhagen.

NOMESCO (2007), *Health Statistics in the Nordic Countries 2005*, NOMESCO, Copenhagen.

OECD (1985), *Measuring Health Care, 1960-1983: Expenditure, Costs and Performance*, OECD Publishing, Paris.

OECD (2000), *A System of Health Accounts*, OECD Publishing, Paris.

OECD (2003a), *A Disease-based Comparison of Health Systems: What is Best and at What Cost?*, OECD Publishing, Paris.

OECD (2003b), *OECD Reviews of Health Care Systems – Korea*, OECD Publishing, Paris.

OECD (2004a), "Monitoring and Improving the Technical Quality of Medical Care: A New Challenge for Policy Makers in OECD Countries", *Towards High-Performing Health Systems: Policy Studies*, OECD Publishing, Paris.

OECD (2004b), *Private Health Insurance in OECD Countries*, OECD Publishing, Paris.

OECD (2004c), *Towards High-Performing Health Systems*, OECD Publishing, Paris.

OECD (2005a), *Long-term Care for Older People*, OECD Publishing, Paris.

OECD (2005b), *OECD Reviews of Health Systems – Finland*, OECD Publishing, Paris.

OECD (2005c), *OECD Reviews of Health Systems – Mexico*, OECD Publishing, Paris.

OECD (2007a), "Immigrant Health Workers in OECD Countries in the Broader Context of Highly Skilled Migration", *International Migration Outlook 2007*, OECD Publishing, Paris.

OECD (2007b), *OECD Regions at a Glance 2007*, OECD Publishing, Paris.

OECD (2007c), "Patient Safety Data Systems in the OECD: A Report of a Joint Irish Department of Health – OECD Conference", *www.oecd.org/dataoecd/12/4/38705981.pdf*.

OECD (2007d), *Pensions at a Glance – Public Policies across OECD Countries*, OECD Publishing, Paris.

OECD (2008a), *OECD Economic Surveys: Czech Republic*, OECD Publishing, Paris.

OECD (2008b), *OECD Economic Surveys: Denmark*, OECD Publishing, Paris.

OECD (2008c), *OECD Economic Surveys: United States*, OECD Publishing, Paris.

OECD (2008d), *Pharmaceutical Pricing Policies in a Global Market*, OECD Publishing, Paris.

OECD (2008e), *The Looming Crisis in the Health Workforce: How Can OECD Countries Respond?*, OECD Publishing, Paris.

OECD (2009a), *Doing Better for Children*, OECD Publishing, Paris.

OECD (2009b), *OECD Economic Outlook*, OECD Publishing, Paris, June.

OECD (2009c), *OECD Economic Surveys: Greece*, OECD Publishing, Paris.

OECD (2009d), *OECD Economic Surveys: United Kingdom*, OECD Publishing, Paris.

OECD (2009e), *OECD Regions at a Glance 2009*, OECD Publishing, Paris.

OECD (2009f), *OECD Health Data 2009 – Statistics and Indicators for 30 Countries*, online and on CD-Rom, OECD Publishing, Paris.

OECD and the World Bank (2008), *OECD Reviews of Health Systems-Turkey*, OECD Publishing, Paris.

OECD and WHO (2006), *OECD Reviews of Health Systems – Switzerland*, OECD Publishing, Paris.

OECD and WHO (2009), "International Migration of Health Workers", Joint OECD-WHO Policy Brief, OECD, Paris.

OECD/International Transport Forum (ITF) (2008), *Trends in the Transport Sector 1970-2006*, OECD/ITF, Paris.

Office of Management and Budget (2009), "A New Era of Responsibility – The 2010 Budget", Washington DC.

Ohmi, H., K. Hirooka, A. Hata and Y. Mochizuki (2001), "Recent Trend of Increase in Proportion of Low Birth Weight Infants in Japan", *International Journal of Epidemiology*, Vol. 30, pp. 1269-1271.

Ollendorf, D.A. et al. (1998), "Potential Economic Benefits of Lower-Extremity Amputation Prevention Strategies in Diabetes", Diabetes Care, Vol. 21, No. 8, pp. 1240-1245.

ONS – Osservatorio Nazionale Screening (2008), *The National Centre for Screening Monitoring*, Sixth Report, ONS, Firenze.

Or, Z. (2000), "Exploring the Effects of Health Care on Mortality Across OECD Countries", Labour Market and Social Policy Occasional Paper, No. 46, OECD Publishing, Paris.

Or, Z., F. Jusot and E. Yilmaz (2008), "Impact of Health Care System on Socioeconomic Inequalities in Doctor Use", IRDES Working Paper, No. 17, Paris.

Orosz, E. and D. Morgan (2004), "SHA-Based National Health Accounts in Thirteen OECD Countries: A Comparative Analysis", OECD Health Working Paper, No. 16, OECD Publishing, Paris.

Parikh, N.I. et al. (2009), "Long-Term Trends in Myocardial Infarction Incidence and Case Fatality in the National Heart, Lung, and Blood Institute's Framingham Heart Study", *Circulation*, pp. 1203-1210, 10 March.

Peden, M. et al. (eds.) (2004), *World Report on Road Traffic Injury Prevention*, World Health Organisation, Geneva.

Petersen, P.E. (2008), "World Health Organization Global Policy for Improvement of Oral Health-World Health Assembly 2007", *International Dental Journal*, Vol. 58, pp. 115-121.

Poos, M.J.J.C. et al. (2008), *Cost of Illness in the Netherlands 2005*, RIVM, Bilthoven.

PHAC – Public Health Agency of Canada (2008), *Organized Breast Cancer Screening Programs in Canada*, Report on Program Performance in 2003 and 2004, PHAC, Canada.

Public Health Agency of Canada (2009), "Publicly Funded Immunization Programs in Canada – Routine Schedule for Infants and Children", *www.phac-aspc.gc.ca/im/ptimprog-progimpt/table-1-eng.php*.

Ram, F.S., J.A. Wedzicha *et al.* (2004), "Hospital at Home for Patients with Acute Exacerbations of Chronic Obstructive Pulmonary Disease: Systematic Review of Evidence", *British Medical Journal*, Vol. 329, pp. 315-320.

Rasmussen, M. *et al.* (2006), "Determinants of Fruit and Vegetable Consumption among Children and Adolescents: A Review of the Literature. Part 1: Quantitative Studies", *International Journal of Behavioral Nutrition and Physical Activity*, Vol. 3, No. 22.

Raymond, I., F. Pedersen *et al.* (2003), "Prevalence of Impaired Left Ventricular Systolic Function and Heart Failure in a Middle-Aged and Elderly Urban Population Segment of Copenhagen", *Heart*, Vol. 89, No. 12, pp. 1422-1429.

Rehm, J. *et al.* (2009), "Global Burden of Disease and Injury and Economic Cost Attributable to Alcohol Use and Alcohol-use Disorder", *The Lancet*, Vol. 373, pp. 2223-2233.

Retzlaff-Roberts, D., C. Chang and R. Rubin (2004), "Technical Efficiency in the Use of Health Care Resources: A Comparison of OECD Countries", *Health Policy*, Vol. 69, pp. 55-72.

RIVM – National Institute for Public Health and the Environment (2008), *Dutch Health Care Performance Report*, Bilthoven.

Sachs, B.P., C. Kobelin, M.A. Castro and F. Frigoletto (1999), "The Risks of Lowering the Cesarean-delivery Rate", *New England Journal of Medicine*, Vol. 340, pp. 54-57.

Sandvik, C. *et al.* (2005), "Personal, Social and Environmental Factors Regarding Fruit and Vegetable Consumption Intake among Schoolchildren in Nine European Countries", *Annals of Nutrition and Metabolism*, Vol. 49, No. 4, pp. 255-266.

Sant, M. *et al.* (2009), " EUROCARE-4. Survival of Cancer Patients Diagnosed in 1995-1999. Results and Commentary", *European Journal of Cancer*, Vol. 45, No. 6, pp. 931-991.

Sarti, C. *et al.* (2003), "Are Changes in Mortality from Stroke Cause by Changes in Stroke Event Rates or Case Fatality? Results from the WHO MONICA Project", *Stroke*, Vol. 34, pp. 1833-1840.

Sassi, F., M. Devaux, J. Church, M. Cecchini and F. Borgonovi (2009a), "Education and Obesity in Four OECD Countries", OECD Health Working Paper, No. 46, OECD Publishing, Paris.

Sassi, F., M. Devaux, M. Cecchini and E. Rusticelli (2009b), "The Obesity Epidemic: Analysis of Past and Projected Future Trends in Selected OECD Countries", OECD Health Working Paper, No. 45, OECD Publishing, Paris.

Sears, M.R. *et al.* (2003), "A Longitudinal, Population-based Cohort Study of Childhood Asthma Followed to Adulthood", *N Engl J Med*, Vol. 349, No. 15, pp. 1414-1422.

Secretary of State for Health (2002), *Delivering the NHS Plan: Next Steps on Investment, Next Steps on Reform*, The Stationery Office, London.

Seenan, P., M. Long and P. Langhorne (2007), "Stroke Units in Their Natural Habitat: Systematic Review of Observational Studies", *Stroke*, Vol. 38, pp. 1886-1892.

SEER – Surveillance, Epidemiology, and End Results Program (2009), *Cancer Statistics Review, 1975-2006*, National Cancer Institute, *www.seer.cancer.gov*, accessed August 18, 2009.

Shafey, O. *et al.* (eds.) (2009), *The Tobacco Atlas*, 3rd edition, American Cancer Society, Atlanta.

Shield, M. (2004), "Addressing Nurse Shortages: What Can Policy Makers Learn from the Econometric Evidence on Nurse Labour Supply?", *The Economic Journal*, Vol. 114, pp. F464-F498.

Siciliani, L. and J. Hurst (2003), "Explaining Waiting Times Variations for Elective Surgery across OECD Countries", OECD Health Working Paper, No. 7, OECD Publishing, Paris.

Simoens, S. and J. Hurst (2006), "The Supply of Physician Services in OECD Countries", OECD Health Working Paper, No. 21, OECD Publishing, Paris.

Singleton, J.A. *et al.* (2000), "Influenza, Pneumococcal, and Tetanus Toxoid Vaccination of Adults – United States, 1993-1997", *Morbidity and Mortality Weekly Report*, Vol. 49, No. SS-9, pp. 39-63.

Smith-Bindman, R., D.L. Miglioretti and E.B. Larson (2008), "Rising Use of Diagnostic Medical Imaging in a Large Inegrated Health System", Health Affairs, Vol. 27, No. 6, pp. 1491-1502.

Society of Obstetricians and Gynaecologists of Canada *et al.* (2008), "Joint Policy Statement on Normal Childbirth", *Journal of Obstetrics and Gynaecology Canada*, Vol. 30, No. 12, pp. 1163-1165.

SOLVD Investigators (1991), "Effect of Enalapril on Survival in Patients with Reduced Left Ventricular Ejection Fractions and Congestive Heart Failure", *New England Journal of Medicine*, Vol. 325, pp. 293-302.

Starfield, B. *et al.* (2005), "Contribution of Primary Care to Health Systems and Health", *The Milbank Quarterly*, Vol. 83, No. 3, pp. 457-502.

Stroke Unit Trialists' Collaboration (1997), "How Do Stroke Units Improve Patient Outcomes? A Collaborative Systematic Review of the Randomized Trials", *Stroke*, Vol. 28, No. 11, pp. 2139-2144.

Swedish Association of Local Authorities and Regions and National Board of Health and Welfare (2008), *Quality and Efficiency in Swedish Health Care – Regional Comparisons 2008*, Stockholm.

Szucs, T. (2004), "Medical Economics in the Field of Influenza: Past, Present and Future", *Virus Research*, Vol. 103, pp. 25-30.

Taggart, D. (2009), "PCI or CABG in Coronary Artery Disease?", *The Lancet*, Vol. 373, pp. 1190-1197.

Taylor, R., K. Arnett and S. Begg (2008), *BreastScreen Aotearoa, Independent Monitoring Report January-June, 2007*, School of Population Health, University of Queensland, Brisbane.

Thompson, D. and A.M. Wolf (2001), "The Medical-Care Burden of Obesity", *Obesity Reviews*, No. 2, International Association for the Study of Obesity, pp. 189-197.

Tisdalea, J.E., M.B. Huang and C. Borzak (2004), "Risk Factors for Hypertensive Crisis: Importance of Out-Patient Blood Pressure Control", *Family Practice*, Vol. 21, pp. 420-424.

Tu, J.V. *et al.* (2009), "National Trends in Rates of Death and Hospital Admissions Related to Acute Myocardial Infarction, Heart Failure and Stroke, 1994-2004", *CMAJ*, Vol. 180, No. 13, pp. E118-E125.

Tunstall-Pedoe, H. (2003), "MONICA's Quarter Century", *European Journal of Cardiovascular Prevention and Rehabilitation*, Vol. 10, No. 6, pp. 409-410.

Tuomilehto, J. *et al.* (2001), "Prevention of Type 2 Diabetes Mellitus by Changes in Lifestyle Among Subjects with Impaired Glucose Tolerance", *New England Journal of Medicine*, Vol. 344, pp. 1343-1350.

UNAIDS – Joint United Nations Programme in HIV/AIDS (2008), *Report on the Global HIV/AIDS Epidemic 2008*, UNAIDS, Geneva.

UNICEF and WHO (2004), *Low Birthweight: Country, Regional and Global Estimates*, UNICEF, New York.

USITC – United States International Trade Commission (2009), *Recent Trends in US Services Trade – 2009 Annual Report*, Publication No. 4084, USITC, Washington DC.

USPSTF – US Preventive Services Task Force (2008), "Screening for Colorectal Cancer: US Preventive Services Task Force Recommendation Statement", *Ann Int Med*, Vol. 149, pp. 627-637.

USRDS – US Renal Data System (2008), *2008 Annual Data Report: Atlas of Chronic Kidney Disease and End-Stage Renal Disease in the United States*, National Institute of Diabetes and Digestive and Kidney Diseases, Bethesda, MD.

van Doorslaer, E. *et al.* (2004), "Income-related Inequality in the Use of Medical Care in 21 OECD Countries", *OECD Health Working Paper*, No. 14, OECD Publishing, May.

van Doorslaer, E. *et al.* (2008), "Horizontal Inequities in Australia's Mixed Public/Private Health Care System", *Health Policy*, Vol. 86, pp. 97-108.

Verdecchia, A. *et al.* (2007), "Recent Cancer Survival in Europe: A 2000-02 Period Analysis of EUROCARE-4 Data", *The Lancet Oncology*, Vol. 8, pp. 784-796.

Villar, J. *et al.* (2006), "Caesarean Delivery Rates and Pregnancy Outcomes: The 2005 WHO Global Survey on Maternal and Perinatal Health in Latin America", *The Lancet*, Vol. 367, pp. 1819-1829.

Vogler, S. *et al.* (2008), "Pharmaceutical Pricing and Reimbursement Information (PPRI) Report", Report Commissioned by the European Commission (DG Sanco) and the Austrian Federal Ministry of Health, Family and Youth, Vienna.

Wahlgren, N. *et al.* (2007), "Thrombolysis with Alteplase for Acute Ischaemic Stroke in the Safe Implementation of Thrombolysis in Stroke-Monitoring Study (SITS-MOST): An Observational Study", *The Lancet*, Vol. 369, pp. 275-282.

Wardlaw, J.M., P.A.G. Sandercock and E. Berge (2003), "Thrombolytic Therapy with Recombinant Tissue Plasminogen Activator for Acute Ischemic Stroke. Where Do We Go From Here? A Cumulative Meta-Analysis", *Stroke*, Vol. 34, pp. 1437-1443.

Wedzicha, J.A. and T.A.R. Seemungal (2007), "COPD Exacerbations: Defining their Cause and Prevention", *The Lancet*, Vol. 370, pp. 786-796.

Weisfeldt, M.L. and S.J. Zieman (2007), "Advances in the Prevention and Treatment of Cardiovascular Disease", *Health Affairs*, Vol. 26, pp. 25-37.

Westert, G.P. *et al.* (ed.) (2008), "Dutch Health Care Performance Report 2008", RIVM National Institute for Public Health and the Environment, Bilthoven.

WHO – World Health Organisation (1996), *Health Behaviour in School-aged Children: A World Health Organisation Cross-national Study (1993/94)*, WHO Regional Office for Europe, Copenhagen.

WHO (2000), "Obesity: Preventing and Managing the Global Epidemic. Report of a WHO Consultation", WHO Technical Report Series No. 894, WHO, Geneva.

WHO (2001), "Mental Health: New Understanding, New Hope", *World Health Report 2001*, WHO, Geneva.

WHO (2002), *World Health Report 2002*, WHO, Geneva.

WHO (2003), *The World Oral Health Report 2003: Continuous Improvement of Oral Health in the 21st Century – The Approach of the WHO Global Oral Health Programme*, WHO, Geneva.

WHO (2004a), "Hepatitis B Vaccines", *Weekly Epidemiological Record*, No. 28, pp. 253-264.

WHO (2004b), *WHO Global Status Report on Alcohol 2004*, WHO, Geneva.

WHO (2005), "World Diabetes Day: Too Many People Are Losing Lower Limbs Unnecessarily to Diabetes", *Joint WHO/International Diabetes Federation News Release*, 11 November 2005, Geneva.

WHO (2006), *Health Statistics and Health Information Systems. Projections of Mortality and Burden of Disease to 2030*, WHO, *www.who.int/healthinfo/global_burden_disease/en/index.html*.

WHO (2008a), *World Alliance for Patient Safety Forward Programme 2008-2009*, First Edition, WHO, Geneva.

WHO (2008b), *World Health Statistics 2008*, WHO, Geneva.

WHO (2009a), *Hepatitis B WHO Fact Sheet No. 204*, WHO, Geneva.

WHO (2009b), *Vaccines for pandemic influenza A (H1N1)*, *www.who.int/csr/disease/swineflu/frequently_asked_questions/vaccine_preparedness/en/index.html*.

WHO (2009c), *Global Status Report on Road Safety: Time for Action*, WHO, Geneva.

WHO Europe (2007), "Prevalence of Excess Body Weight and Obesity in Children and Adolescents", *Fact Sheet No.2.3*, European Environment and Health Information System.

Woods, L.M., B. Rachet and M.P. Coleman (2006), "Origins of Socio-economic Inequalities in Cancer Survival: A Review", *Annals of Oncology*, Vol. 17, No. 1, pp. 5-19.

World Bank (1999), *Curbing the Epidemic: Governments and the Economics of Tobacco Control*, World Bank, Washington.

Xu, K. *et al.* (2007), "Protecting Households From Catastrophic Health Spending", *Health Affairs*, Vol. 26, pp. 972-983.

ANNEX A

Additional Information on Demographic and Economic Context, Health System Characteristics, and Health Expenditure and Financing

Table A.1. **Total population, mid-year, thousands, 1960 to 2007**

	1960	1970	1980	1990	2000	2007
Australia	10 275	12 507	14 695	17 065	19 153	21 017
Austria	7 047	7 467	7 549	7 718	8 110	8 315
Belgium	9 153	9 656	9 859	9 967	10 251	10 623
Canada	17 870	21 297	24 516	27 698	30 689	32 976
Czech Republic	9 660	9 805	10 327	10 362	10 272	10 323
Denmark	4 581	4 929	5 123	5 141	5 340	5 457
Finland	4 430	4 606	4 779	4 986	5 176	5 289
France	45 684	50 772	53 880	56 709	59 049	61 707
Germany[1]	55 585	60 651	61 566	63 254	82 160	82 257
Greece	8 327	8 793	9 642	10 089	10 917	11 193
Hungary	9 984	10 338	10 711	10 374	10 211	10 056
Iceland	176	205	228	255	281	311
Ireland	2 834	2 950	3 401	3 503	3 790	4 339
Italy	48 967	52 771	55 657	56 737	57 189	58 880
Japan	93 419	103 720	117 060	123 611	126 926	127 771
Korea	25 012	32 241	38 124	42 869	47 008	48 456
Luxembourg	315	340	365	384	436	476
Mexico	. .	50 785	67 384	83 971	98 439	105 791
Netherlands	11 486	13 039	14 150	14 951	15 926	16 382
New Zealand	2 377	2 820	3 144	3 363	3 858	4 228
Norway	3 585	3 879	4 086	4 241	4 491	4 709
Poland	29 561	32 526	35 578	38 031	38 256	38 121
Portugal	9 077	8 663	9 819	9 873	10 229	10 604
Slovak Republic	3 994	4 528	4 984	5 298	5 401	5 398
Spain	30 256	33 859	37 527	38 851	40 264	44 873
Sweden	7 480	8 043	8 311	8 559	8 872	9 148
Switzerland	5 328	6 181	6 319	6 712	7 184	7 550
Turkey	27 506	35 321	44 439	56 156	67 420	70 586
United Kingdom	52 373	55 632	56 330	57 237	58 886	60 975
United States	180 671	205 052	227 225	249 623	282 194	301 621
OECD	**717 013**	**853 376**	**946 778**	**1 027 588**	**1 128 378**	**1 179 432**

1. Note that population figures for Germany prior to 1991 refer to West Germany.
⏐ Break in series.
Source: OECD Health Data 2009.

StatLink ᴍᴤ⌐ *http://dx.doi.org/10.1787/720511520030*

Table A.2. **Share of the population aged 65 and over, 1960 to 2007**

	1960	1970	1980	1990	2000	2007
Australia	8.5	8.3	9.6	11.1	12.4	13.1
Austria	12.2	14.1	15.4	15.1	15.5	17.0
Belgium	12.0	13.4	14.3	14.9	16.8	17.1
Canada	7.6	8.0	9.4	11.3	12.6	13.4
Czech Republic	9.6	12.1	13.5	12.5	13.8	14.5
Denmark	10.6	12.3	14.4	15.6	14.8	15.5
Finland	7.3	9.1	12.0	13.4	14.9	16.5
France	11.6	12.9	13.9	14.1	16.1	16.4
Germany	10.8	13.2	15.5	15.3	17.2	20.2
Greece	8.1	11.1	13.1	14.0	16.6	18.6
Hungary	9.0	11.5	13.4	13.4	15.1	16.1
Iceland	8.1	8.9	9.9	10.6	11.6	11.5
Ireland	10.9	11.2	10.7	11.4	11.2	10.8
Italy	9.0	10.5	12.9	14.6	17.7	19.7
Japan	5.7	7.1	9.1	12.1	17.4	21.5
Korea	2.9	3.1	3.8	5.1	7.2	9.9
Luxembourg	10.8	12.6	13.6	13.4	14.1	14.0
Mexico	. .	4.6	4.3	4.1	4.7	5.5
Netherlands	9.0	10.2	11.5	12.8	13.6	14.6
New Zealand	8.7	8.4	9.7	11.1	11.8	12.5
Norway	10.9	12.9	14.8	16.3	15.2	14.6
Poland	5.8	8.2	10.1	10.1	12.2	13.4
Portugal	. .	9.1	11.4	13.6	16.4	17.3
Slovak Republic	6.9	9.2	10.5	10.3	11.4	11.9
Spain	8.2	9.6	11.2	13.6	16.8	16.6
Sweden	11.8	13.7	16.3	17.8	17.3	17.4
Switzerland	10.7	11.8	14.3	15.0	15.8	16.3
Turkey	3.5	4.4	4.7	4.5	5.4	7.1
United Kingdom	11.7	13.0	15.0	15.7	15.8	16.0
United States	9.2	9.8	11.3	12.5	12.4	12.6
OECD	**9.0**	**10.1**	**11.7**	**12.5**	**13.8**	**14.7**

Source: OECD Health Data 2009.

StatLink http://dx.doi.org/10.1787/720520270228

Table A.3. **Fertility rate, number of children per woman aged 15-49, 1960 to 2006**

	1960	1970	1980	1990	2000	2006
Australia	3.5	2.9	1.9	1.9	1.8	1.8
Austria	2.7	2.3	1.7	1.5	1.4	1.4
Belgium	2.6	2.3	1.7	1.6	1.7	1.8
Canada	3.9	2.3	1.7	1.7	1.5	1.5
Czech Republic	2.1	1.9	2.1	1.9	1.1	1.3
Denmark	2.5	2.0	1.6	1.7	1.8	1.9
Finland	2.7	1.8	1.6	1.8	1.7	1.8
France	2.7	2.5	2.0	1.8	1.9	2.0
Germany	2.4	2.0	1.6	1.5	1.4	1.3
Greece	2.3	2.4	2.2	1.4	1.3	1.4
Hungary	2.0	2.0	1.9	1.8	1.3	1.4
Iceland	4.3	2.8	2.5	2.3	2.1	2.1
Ireland	3.8	3.9	3.2	2.1	1.9	1.9
Italy	2.4	2.4	1.7	1.4	1.3	1.4
Japan	2.0	2.1	1.8	1.5	1.4	1.3
Korea	6.0	4.5	2.8	1.6	1.5	1.1
Luxembourg	2.3	2.0	1.5	1.6	1.8	1.6
Mexico	7.3	6.8	5.0	3.4	2.7	2.2
Netherlands	3.1	2.6	1.6	1.6	1.7	1.7
New Zealand	4.2	3.2	2.0	2.2	2.0	2.0
Norway	2.9	2.5	1.7	1.9	1.9	1.9
Poland	3.0	2.2	2.3	2.0	1.4	1.3
Portugal	3.1	2.8	2.2	1.6	1.6	1.4
Slovak Republic	3.1	2.4	2.3	2.1	1.3	1.2
Spain	2.9	2.9	2.2	1.4	1.2	1.4
Sweden	2.2	1.9	1.7	2.1	1.6	1.9
Switzerland	2.4	2.1	1.6	1.6	1.5	1.4
Turkey	6.4	5.0	4.6	3.1	2.3	2.2
United Kingdom	2.7	2.4	1.9	1.8	1.6	1.8
United States	3.7	2.5	1.8	2.1	2.1	2.1
OECD	**3.2**	**2.7**	**2.1**	**1.9**	**1.6**	**1.7**

Source: OECD Health Data 2009.

StatLink ⬛⬛⬛ *http://dx.doi.org/10.1787/720534726070*

Table A.4. **GDP per capita in 2007 and average annual growth rates, 1970 to 2007**

	GDP per capita in USD PPP	Average annual growth rate (in real terms)			
	2007	1970-80	1980-90	1990-2000	2000-07
Australia	37 808	1.3	1.4	2.4	2.0
Austria	37 121	3.5	1.9	2.0	1.7
Belgium	35 380	3.2	1.9	1.9	1.5
Canada	38 500	2.6	1.6	1.9	1.6
Czech Republic	24 027	. .	. .	0.3	4.4
Denmark	35 978	1.9	2.0	2.2	1.3
Finland	34 698	3.3	2.6	1.6	2.8
France	32 684	3.0	1.9	1.5	1.1
Germany	34 393	2.7	2.1	0.3	1.2
Greece	28 423	3.6	0.2	1.5	3.9
Hungary	18 754	. .	. .	. .	4.0
Iceland	35 696	5.3	1.6	1.5	2.7
Ireland	45 214	3.3	3.3	6.2	3.6
Italy	30 794	3.2	2.2	1.5	0.7
Japan	33 603	3.2	3.4	1.0	1.5
Korea	24 801	5.4	7.5	5.1	4.2
Luxembourg	59 484	. .	. .	. .	1.5
Mexico	13 989	3.8	−0.1	1.8	1.4
Netherlands	39 213	2.2	1.8	2.5	1.5
New Zealand	27 140	0.7	1.2	1.5	2.1
Norway	53 443	4.1	2.1	3.1	1.7
Poland	16 089	. .	. .	3.7	4.1
Portugal	22 824	3.5	3.2	2.5	0.6
Slovak Republic	20 073	. .	. .	. .	6.2
Spain	31 586	2.6	2.6	2.4	1.8
Sweden	36 632	1.6	1.9	1.6	2.3
Switzerland	40 877	1.0	1.6	0.4	1.1
Turkey	13 604	. .	. .	1.7	4.2
United Kingdom	35 557	1.8	2.6	2.2	2.1
United States	45 559	2.2	2.3	2.0	1.4
OECD	**32 798**	**2.9**	**2.2**	**2.1**	**2.3**

Source: OECD Health Data 2009.

StatLink ᵐˢᴸ *http://dx.doi.org/10.1787/720564056728*

Table A.5. **Basic primary health insurance coverage of selected functions of care, and share of typical costs covered, 2008-09**

	Acute in-patient care	Outpatient primary care and specialist contacts	Pharmaceuticals	Dental care
Australia	No copayment, 100%	Copayment, 76-99%	Copayment, 76-99%	Not covered
Austria	Copayment, 76-99%	No copayment, 100%	Copayment, 76-99%	No copayment, 100%
Belgium	Copayment, 76-99%	Copayment, 76-99%	Copayment, 76-99%	Copayment, 76-99%
Canada	No copayment, 100%	No copayment, 100%	Copayment, 51-75%	Not covered
Czech Republic	Copayment, 76-99%	Copayment, 76-99%	Copayment, 51-75%	Copayment, 1-50%
Denmark	No copayment, 100%	No copayment, 100%	Copayment, 51-75%	Copayment, 1-50%
Finland	Copayment, 76-99%	Copayment, 76-99%	Copayment, 51-75%	Copayment, 76-99%
France	Copayment, 76-99%	Copayment, 51-75%	Copayment, 51-75%	Copayment, 1-50%
Germany	Copayment, ~100%	Copayment, 76-99%	Copayment, 76-99%	Copayment, 76-99%
Greece	Copayment, 76-99%	Copayment, 76-99%	Copayment, 76-99%	Copayment, 1-50%
Hungary	No copayment, 100%	No copayment, 100%	Copayment, 76-99%	Copayment, 100%[1]
Iceland	Copayment, 76-99%	Copayment, 76-99%	Copayment, 76-99%	Copayment, 76-99%
Ireland	No copayment, 100%	No copayment, 100%	n.a.	Not covered
Italy	No copayment, 100%	No copayment, 76-99%	No copayment, 100%	Copayment
Japan	Copayment, 51-75%	Copayment, 51-75%	Copayment, 51-75%	Copayment, 51-75%
Korea	Copayment, 76-99%	Copayment, 51-75%	Copayment, 51-75%	Copayment, 51-75%
Luxembourg	Copayment, 76-99%	Copayment, 76-99%	Copayment, 76-99%	Copayment, 51-75%
Mexico	No copayment, 100%	No copayment, 100%	No copayment, 100%	No copayment, 100%
Netherlands	No copayment, 100%	No copayment, 100%	No copayment, 100%	Copayment, 1-50%
New Zealand	No copayment, 100%	Copayment, 51-75%	Copayment, 76-99%	Not covered
Norway	No copayment, 100%	Copayment, 76-99%	Copayment, 76-99%	Not covered
Poland	No copayment, 100%	No copayment, 100%	Copayment, 51-75%	No copayment, 100%[1]
Portugal	No copayment, 100%	No copayment, 100%	Copayment, 1-50%	No copayment, 1-50%[1]
Slovak Republic	No copayment, 100%	No copayment, 100%	Copayment, 76-99%	Copayment, 51-75%
Spain	No copayment, 100%	No copayment, 100%	Copayment, 76-99%	Not covered
Sweden	Copayment, 76-99%	Copayment, 76-99%	Copayment, 51-75%	Copayment, 1-50%
Switzerland	Copayment, ~100%	Copayment, 76-99%	Copayment, 76-99%	Not covered
Turkey	No copayment, 100%	Copayment, 76-99%	Copayment, 76-99%	No copayment, 100%
United Kingdom	No copayment, 100%	No copayment, 100%	No copayment, 100%	Copayment, 76-99%
United States	n.a.	n.a.	n.a.	n.a.

n.a.: Not available.

1. In some countries, basic dental services are covered in principle by public schemes, but most care occurs in the private sector.

Source: OECD Survey of Health System Characteristics 2008-2009.

StatLink ⟱ http://dx.doi.org/10.1787/720567687370

Table A.6. **Acute care beds in public and private hospitals, 2008-09**

Percentage

	Publically owned hospitals	Not-for-profit privately owned hospitals	For-profit privately owned hospitals
Australia	70	14	16
Austria	73	19	9
Belgium	34	66	–
Canada	100	–	–
Czech Republic	91	–	9
Denmark	100	–	–
Finland	89	–	11
France	66	9	25
Germany	49	36	15
Greece	69	3	28
Hungary	n.a.	n.a.	n.a.
Iceland	100	–	–
Ireland	n.a.	n.a.	n.a.
Italy	82	17	2
Japan	26	74	–
Korea	10	65	25
Luxembourg	68	29	3
Mexico	65	–	35
Netherlands	–	100	–
New Zealand	81	10	10
Norway	99	1	–
Poland	95	–	5
Portugal	86	7	8
Slovak Republic	60	–	40
Spain	74	17	9
Sweden	98	–	2
Switzerland	83	5	13
Turkey	90	–	11
United Kingdom	96	4	–
United States	n.a.	n.a.	n.a.

n.a.: Not available. Rows may not add to 100% due to rounding.

Source: OECD Survey of Health System Characteristics 2008-2009.

StatLink 🔗 *http://dx.doi.org/10.1787/720618730236*

Table A.7. **Predominant mode of payment for physicians in OECD countries**

	Primary care physicians	Out-patient specialists	In-patient specialists
Australia	Fee-for-service	Fee-for-service	Salary
Austria	Fee-for-service/Capitation	Fee-for-service	Salary
Belgium	Fee-for-service	Fee-for-service	n.a.
Canada	Fee-for-service	Fee-for-service	Fee-for-service
Czech Republic	Fee-for-service/Capitation	Fee-for-service/Salary	Salary
Denmark	Fee-for-service/Capitation	Salary	Salary
Finland	Salary	Salary	Salary
France	Fee-for-service	Fee-for-service	Salary
Germany	Fee-for-service	Fee-for-service	Salary
Greece	Salary	Fee-for-service/Salary	Salary
Hungary	Capitation	Salary	n.a.
Iceland	Salary	Fee-for-service	Salary
Ireland	Capitation	Fee-for-service	Salary
Italy	Capitation	Salary	Salary
Japan	Fee-for-service	Fee-for-service	Salary
Korea	Fee-for-service	Fee-for-service/Salary	Fee-for-service/Salary
Luxembourg	Fee-for-service	Fee-for-service	n.a.
Mexico	Salary	Salary	Salary
Netherlands	Fee-for-service/Capitation	n.a.	Fee-for-service
New Zealand	Fee-for-service/Salary	Fee-for-service/Salary	Fee-for-service/Salary
Norway	Fee-for-service/Capitation	Fee-for-service/Salary	Salary
Poland	Capitation	Fee-for-service	n.a.
Portugal	Salary	Salary	n.a.
Slovak Republic	Capitation	n.a.	Salary
Spain	Salary/Capitation	Salary	Salary
Sweden	Salary	Salary	n.a.
Switzerland	Fee-for-service	Fee-for-service	n.a.
Turkey	Fee-for-service/Salary	Fee-for-service/Salary	Fee-for-service/Salary
United Kingdom	Salary/Capitation/Fee-for-service	Salary	Salary
United States	Salary/Capitation/Fee-for-service	Fee-for-service	n.a.

n.a.: Not available.
Source: OECD Survey of Health System Characteristics 2008-2009.

Table A.8. **Total expenditure on health per capita, USD PPP, 1980 to 2007**

	1980	1990	1995	2000	2005	2006	2007
Australia	644	1 203	1 610	2 271	2 983	3 137	
Austria	783	1 618	2 216	2 824	3 472	3 608	3 763
Belgium	643	1 357	1 853	2 377	3 301	3 356e	3 595e
Canada	780	1 738	2 057	2 516	3 464	3 696	3 895
Czech Republic		559	899	980	1 455	1 513	1 626 .
Denmark	896	1 544	1 871	2 378	3 152	3 357	3 512
Finland	571	1 366	1 481	1 853	2 590	2 709	2 840
France	668	1 449	2 101	2 542	3 303	3 423	3 601
Germany	971	1 768	2 275	2 671	3 348	3 464	3 588
Greece	491	853	1 263	1 449	2 352	2 547	2 727
Hungary		577 1991	660	852	1 411	1 457	1 388
Iceland	755	1 666	1 909	2 736	3 304	3 207	3 319
Ireland	513	791	1 203	1 805	2 831	3 001	3 424
Italy		1 359	1 538	2 052	2 536	2 673	2 686
Japan	585	1 125	1 551	1 967	2 474	2 581	
Korea	107	357	525	809	1 296	1 491	1 688
Luxembourg			1 910	2 553	4 021	4 162e	
Mexico		296	386	508	724	777	823
Netherlands	728	1 416	1 798	2 337	3 450e	3 611e	3 837e
New Zealand	509	990	1 245	1 605	2 253	2 435	2 510
Norway	668	1 369	1 862	3 039	4 301	4 507	4 763
Poland		289	411	583	857	920	1 035
Portugal	276	636	1 035	1 509	2 098	2 150	
Slovak Republic			564 1997	603	1 139	1 322	1 555
Spain	363	872	1 193	1 536	2 267	2 466	2 671
Sweden	946	1 596	1 745	2 283	2 958	3 124	3 323
Switzerland	1 017	2 033	2 568	3 217	4 015	4 165	4 417e
Turkey	70	155	173	432	618		
United Kingdom	470	963	1 349	1 833	2 693	2 885	2 992
United States	1 091	2 810	3 748	4 704	6 558	6 933	7 290
OECD average	**632**	**1 170**	**1 500**	**1 961**	**2 707**	**2 843**	**2 984**

| Break in series.
e: Preliminary estimate.
Source: OECD Health Data 2009.

StatLink 🖳📊 *http://dx.doi.org/10.1787/720642511721*

Table A.9. **Public expenditure on health per capita, USD PPP, 1980 to 2007**

	1980	1990	1995	2000	2005	2006	2007
Australia	404	796	1 059	1 524	2 011	2 124	
Austria	539	1 187	1 638	2 169	2 644	2 737	2 875
Belgium[1]			1 317	1 673	2 377	2 426e	2 601e
Canada	590	1 296	1 468	1 770	2 434	2 580	2 726
Czech Republic		545	817	885	1 289	1 332	1 385
Denmark	787	1 277	1 544	1 961	2 639	2 823	2 968
Finland	451	1 105	1 067	1 317	1 903	2 022	2 120
France	535	1 109	1 674	2 018	2 618	2 709	2 844
Germany	764	1 347	1 856	2 128	2 577	2 660	2 758
Greece	273	458	657	870	1 414	1 580	1 646
Hungary		515 1991	554	602	1 020	1 058	980
Iceland	666	1 443	1 602	2 218	2 688	2 628	2 739
Ireland	421	568	865	1 326	2 193	2 326	2 762
Italy		1 080	1 088	1 488	1 933	2 054	2 056
Japan	417	873	1 288	1 598	2 046	2 097	
Korea	22	130	191	363	675	814	927
Luxembourg			1 766	2 280	3 625	3 782e	
Mexico		120	163	236	329	344	372
Netherlands[1]	505	949	1 278	1 474	2 087e	2 731e	2 871e
New Zealand	447	816	961	1 252	1 755	1 898	1 898
Norway	569	1 134	1 569	2 507	3 593	3 776	4 005
Poland		265	299	408	594	643	733
Portugal	178	417	648	1 095	1 505	1 538	
Slovak Republic			517 1997	539	848	903	1 040
Spain	290	687	861	1 100	1 600	1 757	1 917
Sweden	875	1 434	1 512	1 938	2 415	2 548	2 716
Switzerland		1 065	1 375	1 783	2 388	2 463	2 618e
Turkey	21	95	122	272	441		
United Kingdom	420	804	1 132	1 454	2 206	2 367	2 446
United States	445	1 102	1 683	2 033	2 915	3 132	3 307
OECD average	**458**	**838**	**1 086**	**1 409**	**1 959**	**2 076**	**2 176**

1. Public current expenditure.
ı Break in series.
e: Preliminary estimate.
Source: OECD Health Data 2009.

StatLink 🔗 *http://dx.doi.org/10.1787/720660326333*

Table A.10. **Annual growth rate of total expenditure on health per capita, in real terms, 1997 to 2007**

	1997/98	1998/99	1999/2000	2000/01	2001/02	2002/03	2003/04	2004/05	2005/06	2006/07
Australia	4.5[1]	4.9	4.5	4.3	4.4	1.5	4.6	0.9	1.9	
Austria	5.3	4.5	1.7	1.7	2.5	2.1	3.0	1.7	1.4	1.7
Belgium	3.0	5.9	3.9	1.7	3.7	5.1[1]	6.5	2.9[1]	−0.7	3.8
Canada	6.2	3.1	3.6	6.1	5.1	2.9	2.1	2.7	3.4	2.6
Czech Republic	−1.2	0.4	2.8[1]	5.1	8.2	4.6[1]	0.9	5.4	2.6	3.5
Denmark	3.9	4.0	0.7	4.0	2.5	3.1[1]	3.7	2.6	4.4	2.7
Finland	0.9	4.2	2.6	4.7	6.7	6.3	4.6	5.1	2.8	2.1
France	2.1	3.0	2.5	2.4	3.5	3.9	2.8	2.2	0.8	1.5
Germany	2.1	2.7	3.0	2.5	1.7	1.2	−1.0	1.8	1.9	1.5
Greece	2.0	6.0	11.1[1]	16.1	6.5	3.9	0.7	11.8	5.2	4.2
Hungary	3.1[1]	5.0	2.3	7.6	10.5	6.3[1]	2.0	7.7	1.3	−7.3
Iceland	15.7	11.1	1.5	0.8	7.9	4.7[1]	1.5	1.4	−1.7	3.3
Ireland	4.2	9.9	8.4	15.2	7.6	5.0	6.1	1.0	1.2	9.6
Italy	2.2	2.2	7.1	3.4	1.8	0.1	5.1	2.9	2.2	−2.2
Japan	1.9	3.2	4.6	3.3	0.4	2.8	2.1	3.4	1.0	
Korea	−6.0	14.7	15.5	14.9	3.6	7.8	5.2	11.7	11.4	10.3
Luxembourg	5.0	7.9	5.0	7.9	8.7	9.1[1]	9.5	−2.5	−2.3	
Mexico	7.5[1]	6.8	4.5	5.9	2.8	3.2	3.6	2.4	4.0	3.2
Netherlands	2.4[1]	4.3	1.5	5.5	6.3	5.1[1]	3.9	0.4	2.2	3.8
New Zealand	5.6	3.1	2.9	4.4	7.4	0.0	8.4	9.1	3.9	0.9
Norway	12.4	2.2	−7.4	6.1	12.3	2.7	−0.5	−3.9	−3.5	5.2
Poland	10.6	1.5	0.4	7.4	4.9[1]	2.4	4.7	3.8	6.1	12.1
Portugal	1.4	6.9	4.0[1]	1.0	2.0	6.3	3.8	2.3	−1.2	
Slovak Republic	1.9	1.7	−3.2	4.0	7.0	8.3	6.2[1]	4.1	12.9	16.5
Spain	3.9	3.3[1]	2.7	2.9	1.4	1.8[1]	2.1	3.1	3.2	3.0
Sweden	5.3	5.6	4.0	5.0[1]	5.9	2.7	1.4	2.5	2.6	1.9
Switzerland	3.6	2.1	2.5	4.9	2.7	2.2	2.2	1.3	−0.9	2.1
Turkey	16.1	12.6[1]	9.1	4.3	10.5	6.3	7.1	2.7		
United Kingdom	4.1	6.8	5.4	5.3	6.2	5.1	5.9	3.7	4.9	1.9
United States	3.3	3.5	3.5	4.9	6.1	5.1	2.9	2.5	2.4	2.4
OECD average	**4.4**	**5.1**	**3.7**	**5.4**	**5.4**	**4.0**	**3.7**	**3.2**	**2.5**	**3.6**

1. Adjusted rate. See "Definition and deviations" for Indicator 7.1 "Health expenditure per capita".
Source: OECD Health Data 2009.

StatLink ᵐˢᐧ *http://dx.doi.org/10.1787/720666460464*

Table A.11. **Annual growth rate of public expenditure on health per capita, in real terms, 1997 to 2007**

	1997/98	1998/99	1999/2000	2000/01	2001/02	2002/03	2003/04	2004/05	2005/06	2006/07
Australia	7.5[2]	8.2	2.5	2.7	5.5	1.2	5.5	1.4	2.4	
Austria	5.7	5.6	1.8	0.7	2.1	1.8	3.2	2.3	1.1	2.4
Belgium[1]	2.3	5.4	4.1	3.7	0.9	4.4[2]	7.9	3.8[2]	−0.4	3.9
Canada	6.9	2.2	4.1	5.5	4.5	3.9	2.1	2.8	2.7	2.9
Czech Republic	−1.0	0.4	2.5[2]	4.5	9.0	4.6[2]	0.1	4.8	1.9	0.2
Denmark	3.6	4.3	0.9	4.3	2.8	3.1[2]	3.4	2.6	4.9	3.2
Finland	0.3	3.7	2.0	5.9	7.4	6.6	5.3	5.8	4.5	2.1
France	1.9	2.9	2.4	2.4	3.8	3.6	2.7	2.1	0.7	1.3
Germany	1.2	2.3	2.9	2.1	1.6	0.6	−3.2	1.8	1.7	1.6
Greece	0.5	8.8	13.2[2]	17.5	1.7	7.1	−0.4	13.7	8.6	1.4
Hungary	1.3[2]	1.7	0.0	4.9	12.5	7.0[2]	1.4	7.6	1.7	−9.8
Iceland	13.4	13.5	0.1	0.7	9.1	5.0[2]	0.9	1.5	−1.0	4.0
Ireland	4.0	8.9	9.0	16.1	10.2	7.6	6.6	0.2	1.2	14.1
Italy	1.5	2.8	9.8	6.5	1.6	0.1	7.2	3.3	3.0	−2.6
Japan	1.0	3.6	4.9	3.8	0.1	2.8	2.5	4.6	−0.7	
Korea	3.5	16.9	10.8	32.4	1.4	6.0	7.2	14.6	16.8	11.0
Luxembourg	4.9	4.9	4.4	6.2	11.6	10.8[2]	9.9	−2.5	−1.6	
Mexico	13.8[2]	10.9	1.8	2.1	0.5	3.8	8.9	0.4	1.1	5.4
Netherlands[1]	2.5[2]	2.0	2.1	5.0	5.7	3.7[2]	1.6	1.5		2.7
New Zealand	5.3	3.7	3.6	2.3	9.5	0.6	6.9	10.0	4.0	
Norway	13.7	2.6	−7.5	7.4	12.2	3.0	−0.7	−3.9	−3.2	5.6
Poland	0.5	10.4	−1.1	10.3	5.5[2]	0.6	2.7	4.9	7.0	12.2
Portugal	3.6	7.7	3.6[2]	−0.5	3.1	7.8	2.0	1.9	−1.5	
Slovak Republic	1.8	−0.5	−3.5	3.9	6.7	7.4	6.2[2]	5.0	3.7	14.0
Spain	3.5	2.8[2]	2.1	2.3	1.5	1.9[2]	2.3	3.2	4.2	3.8
Sweden	5.2	5.5	3.0	4.6[2]	6.2	3.3	0.5	2.3	2.5	2.0
Switzerland	3.0	3.0	3.0	7.7	4.1	3.3	2.3	3.2	−1.5	2.4
Turkey	16.7	14.5[2]	12.3	13.1	14.0	8.1	8.1	1.4		
United Kingdom	4.1	7.1	3.7	6.2	6.1	5.4	7.8	4.1	5.0	1.5
United States	0.7	2.5	3.8	7.2	5.9	4.7	3.7	2.9	4.1	2.8
OECD average	**4.4**	**5.6**	**3.4**	**6.4**	**5.6**	**4.3**	**3.8**	**3.6**	**2.6**	**3.7**

1. Public current expenditure.
2. Adjusted rate. See "Definition and deviations" for Indicator 7.1 "Health expenditure per capita".
Source: OECD Health Data 2009.

StatLink ⫘⎚ *http://dx.doi.org/10.1787/720670137852*

Table A.12. **Total expenditure on health, percentage of GDP, 1980 to 2007**

	1980	1990	1995	2000	2005	2006	2007
Australia	6.3	6.9	7.4	8.3	8.7	8.7	
Austria	7.4	8.3	9.5	9.9	10.4	10.2	10.1
Belgium	6.3	7.2	8.2	8.6	10.3	10.0e	10.2e
Canada	7.0	8.9	9.0	8.8	9.9	10.0	10.1
Czech Republic		4.7	7.0	6.5	7.1	6.9	6.8
Denmark	8.9	8.3	8.1	8.3	9.5	9.6	9.8
Finland	6.3	7.7	7.9	7.2	8.5	8.3	8.2
France	7.0	8.4	10.4	10.1	11.1	11.0	11.0
Germany	8.4	8.3	10.1	10.3	10.7	10.5	10.4
Greece	5.9	6.6	8.6	7.9	9.4	9.5	9.6
Hungary		7.0 1991	7.3	6.9	8.3	8.1	7.4
Iceland	6.3	7.8	8.2	9.5	9.4	9.1	9.3
Ireland	8.3	6.1	6.7	6.3	7.3	7.1	7.6
Italy		7.7	7.3	8.1	8.9	9.0	8.7
Japan	6.5	6.0	6.9	7.7	8.2	8.1	
Korea	4.1	4.3	4.1	4.9	6.1	6.5	6.8
Luxembourg	5.2	5.4	5.6	5.8	7.7	7.3e	
Mexico		4.4	5.1	5.1	5.8	5.8	5.9
Netherlands	7.4	8.0	8.3	8.0	9.8e	9.7e	9.8e
New Zealand	5.9	6.9	7.2	7.7	9.1	9.4	9.2
Norway	7.0	7.6	7.9	8.4	9.1	8.6	8.9
Poland		4.8	5.5	5.5	6.2	6.2	6.4
Portugal	5.3	5.9	7.8	8.8	10.2	9.9	
Slovak Republic			5.8 1997	5.5	7.0	7.3	7.7
Spain	5.3	6.5	7.4	7.2	8.3	8.4	8.5
Sweden	8.9	8.2	8.0	8.2	9.2	9.1	9.1
Switzerland	7.3	8.2	9.6	10.2	11.2	10.8	10.8e
Turkey	2.4	2.7	2.5	4.9	5.7		
United Kingdom	5.6	5.9	6.8	7.0	8.2	8.5	8.4
United States	9.0	12.2	13.6	13.6	15.7	15.8	16.0
OECD average	**6.6**	**6.9**	**7.6**	**7.8**	**8.9**	**8.8**	**8.9**

| Break in series.
e: Preliminary estimate.
Source: OECD Health Data 2009.

StatLink 🔗 *http://dx.doi.org/10.1787/720674486382*

Table A.13. **Public expenditure on health, percentage of GDP, 1980 to 2007**

	1980	1990	1995	2000	2005	2006	2007
Australia	3.9	4.6	4.9	5.6	5.9	5.9	
Austria	5.1	6.1	7.0	7.6	7.9	7.8	7.7
Belgium[1]			5.8	6.1	7.4	7.2e	7.4e
Canada	5.3	6.6	6.4	6.2	7.0	7.0	7.1
Czech Republic		4.6	6.4	5.9	6.3	6.1	5.8
Denmark	7.9	6.9	6.7	6.8	7.9	8.1	8.2
Finland	5.0	6.2	5.7	5.1	6.2	6.2	6.1
France	5.6	6.4	8.3	8.0	8.8	8.7	8.7
Germany	6.6	6.3	8.2	8.2	8.2	8.1	8.0
Greece	3.3	3.5	4.5	4.7	5.7	5.9	5.8
Hungary		6.3 1991	6.1	4.9	6.0	5.9	5.2
Iceland	5.5	6.8	6.9	7.7	7.7	7.5	7.7
Ireland	6.8	4.4	4.8	4.6	5.6	5.5	6.1
Italy		6.1	5.1	5.8	6.8	6.9	6.7
Japan	4.7	4.6	5.7	6.2	6.7	6.6	
Korea	0.8	1.6	1.5	2.2	3.2	3.5	3.7
Luxembourg	4.8	5.0	5.1	5.2	6.9	6.6e	
Mexico		1.8	2.2	2.4	2.7	2.6	2.7
Netherlands[1]	5.1	5.4	5.9	5.0	5.9e	7.4e	7.3e
New Zealand	5.2	5.7	5.5	6.0	7.1	7.3	7.3
Norway	5.9	6.3	6.6	6.9	7.6	7.2	7.5
Poland		4.4	4.0	3.9	4.3	4.3	4.6
Portugal	3.4	3.8	4.9	6.4	7.3	7.1	
Slovak Republic			5.3 1997	4.9	5.2	5.0	5.2
Spain	4.2	5.1	5.4	5.2	5.8	6.0	6.1
Sweden	8.2	7.4	6.9	7.0	7.5	7.4	7.4
Switzerland		4.3	5.1	5.6	6.7	6.4	6.4e
Turkey	0.7	1.6	1.8	3.1	4.1		
United Kingdom	5.0	4.9	5.7	5.6	6.7	6.9	6.9
United States	3.7	4.8	6.1	5.9	7.0	7.1	7.3
OECD average	**4.9**	**5.1**	**5.5**	**5.6**	**6.4**	**6.4**	**6.4**

1. Public current expenditure.
I Break in series.
e: Preliminary estimate.
Source: OECD Health Data 2009.

StatLink 📊 *http://dx.doi.org/10.1787/720674638627*

ANNEX B

List of Variables in OECD Health Data 2009

Part 1. Health status

Mortality
  Life expectancy
  Causes of mortality
  Maternal and infant mortality
  Potential years of life lost
Morbidity
  Perceived health status
  Infant health
  Dental health
  Communicable diseases (HIV/AIDS)
  Cancer
  Injuries
  Absence from work due to illness

Part 2. Health care resources

Health education
Health employment
  Total health and hospital employment
  Physicians
  Midwives and nurses
  Other health professions (dentists and pharmacists)
Remuneration of health professionals
Hospital beds
Medical technology

Part 3. Health care utilisation

Prevention (immunisation)
Screening
Diagnostic exams
Consultations (doctors and dentists)
Average length of stay in hospitals by diagnostic categories
Hospital discharges by diagnostic categories
Surgical procedures
  Total surgical procedures
  Surgical procedures by categories
  Transplants and dialyses

Part 4. Long-term care resources and utilisation

Long-term care beds in institutions
Long-term care workers
Long-term care recipients in institutions and at home

Part 5. Expenditure on health

Total and current expenditure on health
  Investment on medical facilities
Expenditure on personal health care
  Expenditure on medical services
  Expenditure on in-patient care
  Expenditure on day care
  Expenditure on out-patient care
  Expenditure on home care
  Expenditure on ancillary services
  Expenditure on medical goods
  Pharmaceuticals and other medical non-durables
  Therapeutic appliances and other medical durables

Expenditure on collective health care
  Expenditure on prevention and public health
  Expenditure on health administration and insurance
Additional health expenditure aggregates
  Preventive-curative health care
  Total long-term care expenditure
  Total current health and LTC expenditure
Current health expenditure by provider
  Expenditure on hospital services
  Exp. on services of nursing qnd residential care facilities
  Exp. on services of ambulatory health care providers
  Exp. for retail sale and other providers of medical goods
  Exp. on services of public health organisations
  Exp. on services of health care administration
  Exp. on health services of other industries and rest of world
Expenditure by age and gender
Price index

Part 6. Health care financing

Health expenditure by financing agent/scheme
  General government revenues
  Social security schemes
  Out-of-pocket payments
  Private insurance

Part 7. Social protection

Social expenditure
Health care coverage
  Government/social health insurance
  Private health insurance

Part 8. Pharmaceutical market

Pharmaceutical industry activity
Pharmaceutical consumption by selected drugs
Pharmaceutical sales by selected drugs

Part 9. Non-medical determinants of health

Life styles and behaviour
  Food consumption
  Alcohol consumption
  Tobacco consumption
  Body weight and composition
Environment: air quality

Part 10. Demographic references

General demographics
Population age structure

Part 11. Economic references

Macroeconomic references
Monetary conversion rates

Other tables

Satisfaction with health care systems

More information on *OECD Health Data 2009* is available at *www.oecd.org/health/healthdata*.

OECD PUBLISHING, 2, rue André-Pascal, 75775 PARIS CEDEX 16
PRINTED IN FRANCE
(81 2009 11 1 P) ISBN 978-92-64-06153-8 – No. 56967 2009